From Pathophysiology to Treatment of Huntington's Disease

Edited by Natalia Szejko

Published in London, United Kingdom

From Pathophysiology to Treatment of Huntington's Disease
http://dx.doi.org/10.5772/intechopen.94806
Edited by Natalia Szejko

Contributors
Liam Chen, Taylor G. Brown, Elisabeth Petrasch-Parwez, Constanze Rana Parwez, Sarah Maria Von Hein, Carsten Saft, Hans-Werner Habbes, Marlen Löbbecke-Schumacher, Irina Kerkis, Rodrigo Pinheiro Araldi, Cristiane Valverde Wenceslau, Thais Biude Mendes, Nadine van de Zande, Susanne de Bot, Jeroen de Bresser, Eidrees Ghariq, Natalia Szejko, Kamila Saramak, Saravanan Jayaram, Praveen Thaggikuppe Krishnamurthy, Meghana Joshi, Vishnu Kumar, Omar Deeb, Afnan Atallah, Sawsan Salameh

First published in London, United Kingdom, 2022 by IntechOpen
IntechOpen is the global imprint of INTECHOPEN LIMITED, registered in England and Wales, registration number: 11086078, 5 Princes Gate Court, London, SW7 2QJ, United Kingdom

British Library Cataloguing-in-Publication Data
A catalogue record for this book is available from the British Library

Additional hard and PDF copies can be obtained from orders@intechopen.com

From Pathophysiology to Treatment of Huntington's Disease
Edited by Natalia Szejko
p. cm.
Print ISBN 978-1-80355-426-6
Online ISBN 978-1-80355-427-3
eBook (PDF) ISBN 978-1-80355-428-0

Meet the editor

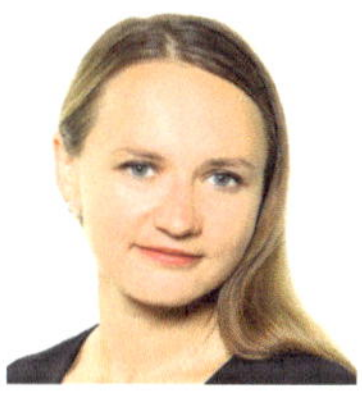

Natalia Szejko, MD, Ph.D., ScD, is an Assistant Professor in the Department of Bioethics at the Medical University of Warsaw and a neurologist in the Department of Neurology at the Medical University of Warsaw. She completed her Ph.D. in 2018 and her ScD in 2020, both at the Medical University of Warsaw. In 2020/2021 she held a postdoctoral fellowship at the Department of Neurology, Yale University, USA. She has complemented her education with a variety of clinical and research fellowships in Germany, Spain, Austria, and the USA. Her main area of interest are movement disorders such as tics, Parkinson's, and Huntington's Disease. She is secretary of the European Society for the Study of Tourette's Syndrome and co-author of the new European guidelines issued by this society, as well as an author of more than 50 publications and book chapters, mainly dedicated to movement disorders.

Contents

Preface **IX**

Section 1
Biomarkers of Huntington's Disease **1**

Chapter 1 **3**
Neuropathology in Huntington's Disease: A Balancing Act between Neurodegeneration and Aggregates
by Elisabeth Petrasch-Parwez, Hans-Werner Habbes, Marlen Löbbecke-Schumacher, Constanze Rana Parwez, Carsten Saft and Sarah Maria von Hein

Chapter 2 **19**
Neuropathology of Huntington's Disease
by Taylor G. Brown and Liam Chen

Chapter 3 **43**
Exploring Biomarkers for Huntington's Disease
by Omar Deeb, Afnan Atallah and Sawsan Salameh

Chapter 4 **65**
Neuroimaging Biomarkers for Huntington's Disease
by Nadine van de Zande, Eidrees Ghariq, Jeroen de Bresser and Susanne de Bot

Section 2
Advances in Treatment of Huntington's Disease **99**

Chapter 5 **101**
Endocannabinoid System as a New Therapeutic Avenue for the Treatment of Huntington's Disease
by Kamila Saramak and Natalia Szejko

Chapter 6 **113**
Advances in Cellular and Cell-Free Therapy Medicinal Products for Huntington Disease Treatment
by Irina Kerkis, Rodrigo Pinheiro Araldi, Cristiane Valverde Wenceslau and Thais Biude Mendes

Chapter 7 **141**
Nrf2 as a Potential Therapeutic Target for Treatment of Huntington's Disease
by Saravanan Jayaram, Praveen Thaggikuppe Krishnamurthy, Meghana Joshi and Vishnu Kumar

Preface

Huntington's Disease (HD) is a neurodegenerative disease caused by the autosomal dominant mutation, in particular, CAG trinucleotide expansion, in the huntingtin gene on chromosome 4. It is characterized by complex phenomenology, in particular, cognitive, motor, and psychiatric symptoms. When it comes to pathophysiology, it has been demonstrated that mutant huntingtin leads to neuronal death via a number of mechanisms such as mitochondrial abnormalities, disruption of protein regulation, and direct toxicity of the mutant protein. Early changes are mainly detected in the striatum, but also the cortex as the disease progresses. In recent years there have been significant advances in research dedicated to HD biomarkers, diagnosis, and, finally, therapy. To date, only symptomatic treatment has been available. With the consequent urgent need for studies to identify new targets for therapeutic interventions, not only is research focused on the development of new treatments of utmost importance, but basic science, neuroimaging and biomarkers are also relevant. With this book, we would like to raise awareness of the most up-to-date HD science. We hope that it will be of use to both experts and the general public.

Natalia Szejko
Department of Neurology,
Department of Bioethics,
Medical University of Warsaw,
Warsaw, Poland

Section 1

Biomarkers of Huntington's Disease

Chapter 1

Neuropathology in Huntington's Disease: A Balancing Act between Neurodegeneration and Aggregates

Elisabeth Petrasch-Parwez, Hans-Werner Habbes, Marlen Löbbecke-Schumacher, Constanze Rana Parwez, Carsten Saft and Sarah Maria von Hein

Abstract

Neuropathology of Huntington's disease (HD) presents with progredient neuronal cell loss mainly in the striatum, but also in multiple other brain areas suggesting HD as a multisystem neurodegenerative disorder. Mutant huntingtin aggregates are the characteristic hallmark of HD. The aggregates are misfolded proteins varying in location, form, size and structural composition indicating a complex involvement in neurotoxicity. The question if and how the aggregates and many interacting protein partners may lead to cell death is continuously a matter of debate. The role of mutant huntingtin is more than ever of paramount importance as present genetic therapeutic approaches try to target downregulation of the Huntingtin gene expression and/or lowering the corresponding protein. In this context—and these aspects are focussed—it is of crucial interest to elucidate the regional distribution as well as the cellular and subcellular localization of aggregates in established animal models of HD and in affected HD brains.

Keywords: Huntington's disease, mutant huntingtin, misfolded proteins, aggregates, inclusion bodies, neurodegeneration, human HD brain, R6/2 mouse, tgHD rat, EM48-immunohistochemistry, transmission electron microscopy

1. Introduction

The autosomal dominantly transmitted Huntington's disease (HD) is caused by an expanded cytosine-adenine-guanine (CAG) trinucleotide repeat in exon 1 of the Huntingtin gene (*HTT*) resulting in an abnormally long polyglutamine tract in the protein huntingtin (Htt; [1]). Patients with 36–39 CAG repeats have an increasing risk to develop HD characteristic symptoms and repeats of 40 and more will result in onset of the disease within a normal lifespan [2]. In about 90% of adult-onset HD patients, the mean age of onset is between 35 and 50 years with marked individual variations; duration of the illness is usually 15–20 years. There is also a correlation between the CAG repeat length and the age of onset in HD [3]. Manifest patients

≤20 years were classified as juvenile-onset HD patients with an estimated prevalence of up to 15%, associated with CAG repeats >60 leading to early death [4, 5]. Core clinical symptoms are cognitive decline, progredient motor impairments and psychiatric alterations—the latter often preceding the onset of the other symptoms.

Neuropathologically, HD shows progredient neuronal cell loss most pronounced in the neostriatum, but also in many other cortical and non-cortical brain areas with considerable regional differences between the HD individuals reflecting the high variability of clinical symptoms. Currently, there is no cure for HD, and only symptoms can be treated.

HD-affected brains show misfolded proteins in form of mutant Huntingtin (mHtt) aggregates, which may be toxic or protective, and their pathomechanism is far from being understood. Aggregates are detected in the nucleus of neurons, the cytoplasm, cell processes and the neuropil. Notably, new therapies address lowering the *mHTT* gene production and/or mHtt protein expression to slow down or even stop disease progression [6, 7]. Therefore, localization of mHtt in HD-affected brains is of major interest in the interplay between the pathogenesis and therapeutic approaches.

In this chapter, we start with some general aspects on neurodegeneration in the human HD brain, then review the distribution and composition of mHtt aggregates and inclusions in two selected rodent models and in human HD brains and conclude with an outlook to future studies to further elucidate the controversial discussion about aggregates and their toxicity.

2. Neurodegeneration in human HD brains

Degeneration of human HD brains has been reported long before the causative gene was detected [8, 9]. The diagnosis was initially performed according to family history, characteristic choreiform movements, cognitive decline and the progredient course of the disease. First post-mortem studies focussed on bilateral striatal atrophy that has always been the most pronounced and consistent macroscopic alteration of the HD brain. The striatal atrophy, which occurs in 95% of all examined HD post-mortem brains, has led to the grading system of Vonsattel, still the most used tool when neurodegeneration of the human HD brain is classified [10, 11]. Based on a high number of post-mortem brains, Vonsattel evaluated the degeneration of striatal areas including the caudate nucleus and putamen as dorsal (motor) and the accumbens as ventral (limbic) neostriatum and the globus pallidus with its external and internal segment as paleostriatum, the latter belonging to the diencephalon. The caudate nucleus and putamen are first affected with a progredient caudo-rostral, medio-lateral and dorso-ventral shift, followed by the accumbens ventrally to the head of the caudate nucleus. Vonsattel determined the temporospatial striatal atrophy into five grades (0–4), also involving the pathohistology of the affected areas. An example of the striatal atrophy at grade 3–4 is documented in **Figure 1A**. At this advanced stage of degeneration, the medial striatal outline bordering the ventricle is straight, the caudate nucleus can hardly be identified and the putamen and globus pallidus are enormously shrunken. The neostriatal atrophy is due to the progredient loss of medium-sized projection neurons that are with about 90–95% the most abundant neuronal cell type in all neostriatal areas (**Figure 1C**). With progredient degeneration, most neurons are dysmorph or lost in the caudate nucleus and putamen, especially in the dorsal parts, accompanied by a marked increase in glial cells (**Figure 1B**). In HD, astrocytosis was reported to be inversely proportional to neuronal cell loss with a later

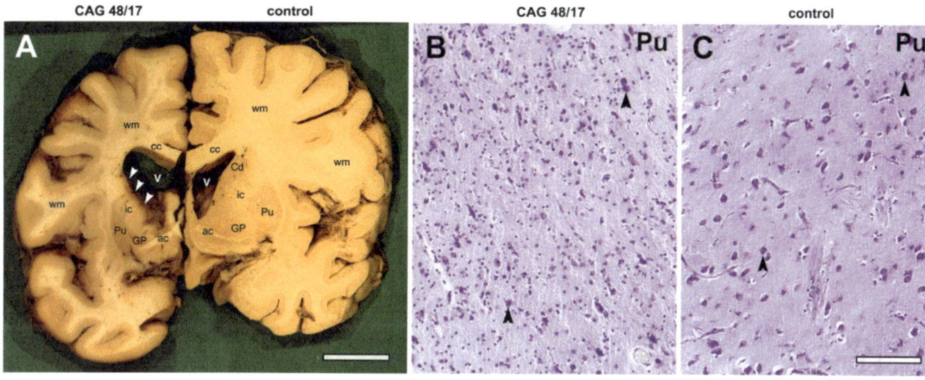

Figure 1.
(A) Frontal HD brain section at advanced degeneration stage (Vonsattel grade 3–4) and a control brain at comparable striatal level with the anterior commissure (ac). Atrophy of the caudate nucleus (Cd) adjacent to the internal capsule (ic) leads to straight outline (white arrowheads) bordering the enlarged lateral ventricle (V) not observed in striatal areas of the control brain. Putamen (Pu) and globus pallidus (GP) also display severe atrophy. Note the shrinkage of white matter (wm) and the corpus callosum (cc) in the HD brain.
(B) Cresyl violet-stained paraffin section (15 µm) of the HD putamen displays loss of most medium-sized striatal neurons with some neuronal cell bodies left (black arrowheads) and a pronounced gliosis as detected by abundant small cell nuclei. (C) Section of the control brain shows normal distribution of medium-sized striatal neurons (black arrowheads). Bar in A = 5 cm; bar in C for B and C = 150 µm.

beginning, whereas the density of oligodendrocytes was already increased at the early Vonsattel grades 0, 1 and 2 [12]. An increase in oligodendrocytes was also observed in the tail of caudate nucleus in HD mutation carriers already prior to the onset of symptoms [13]. A grade-dependant increase of activated microglia was also found in the dorsal neostriatum and globus pallidus [14]. In contrast, ventral striatal areas only show mild neuronal cell loss and moderate gliosis, even at advanced stage of degeneration [11]. The pronounced vulnerability of medium-sized projection neurons is still unclear [15, 16] and the fate of local aspiny striatal interneurons which make up about 5–10% of all striatal neurons is still controversial. They appear to be less and later affected in HD [17]. The striatal interneurons consist of different subpopulations all of which may undergo a different grade-dependant degeneration pattern [18]. Notably, striatal atrophy is also correlated with HD repeat size, younger age of onset and age of death [19].

The globus pallidus as the main neostriatal projection area also undergoes severe atrophy in HD (**Figure 1A**). Pallidal degeneration starts later at Vonsattel grade 2 up to a volume loss of around 50% at grade 4 with the external (the major output target area of the dorsal neostriatum) more affected than the medial segment [20]. Interestingly, the pallidal volume shrinkage is mainly due to loss of neuropil [11, 21], which could represent the reduction of projection axons emerging from neostriatal neurons und their synaptic terminals densely contacting the large pallidal neurons and their proximal dendritic shafts.

Beyond the striatum cortical, other diencephalic and brainstem areas are also affected though highly variable in expression. Morphometric studies of the telencephalon detected that all four lobes showed cortical atrophy more expressed in parietal and occipital than in frontal and temporal areas [22]. These observations were confirmed by MRI-based studies [23]. Imaging studies can be applied in large cohorts of patients in pre-symptomatic, early, middle and late stages and are therefore valuable tools for investigating the development of atrophy in HD brains. A recent MRI study in HD patients carried out annually over a time period of 10 years also confirmed the greatest atrophy in parietal and occipital cortical areas [24]. Remarkably, neuronal cell loss is considerably variable between HD subjects as detected in selected cortical areas [25]. Furthermore, loss of neurons in the primary motor cortex is related to motor symptoms, whereas loss of neurons in the anterior cingulate cortex is related to mood disturbances [26]. To date, many cortical areas have not yet been examined.

In addition to pallidal studies, diencephalic investigations focussed on thalamic and hypothalamic affection. A voxel-based morphometry-based study detected a co-variation between atrophy and cognitive performance suggesting impairment in executive functions [27]. Atrophy is described in the centromedian/parafascicular thalamic complex [28]. The centromedian nucleus is involved into the sensorimotor-associated basal-ganglia-thalamo-cortical feedback loop. The mediodorsal nucleus, which is involved in the corresponding limbic loop, also shows significant neuronal cell loss [29]. Thus, thalamic nuclei involved in HD-associated functionally important feedback loops appear to be severely affected in HD.

Interestingly, the hypothalamus shows a significant loss of grey matter signals already in prodromal HD individuals [30]. Some non-motor dysfunctions are discussed to be associated with changes in neuropeptidergic cell populations disturbing hypothalamic circuitry [31]. Dysfunctions include daily hormone excretion pattern and circadian rhythm disorders, which could also be a target for therapeutic treatment in the disease.

As HD patients show cognitive decline such as planning deficits and short-term memory impairments often already in prodromal phases of the disease, hippocampal involvement should also be considered. A mild but significant atrophy of the hippocampus formation was observed by Lange and Aulich [22] and later confirmed by MRI-based morphometric studies [23]. Accordingly, Vonsattel et al. [11] detected loss of neurons and gliosis in numerous HD cases. However, to really evaluate the hippocampal impact on cognitive impairments, more specific studies on the different subdivisions and cell populations in correlation with clinical symptoms are necessary.

Consistent neuronal loss was also detected in brain stem areas such as substantia nigra, superior and inferior olive, pontine and vestibular nuclei [32]. Regional brain stem affection may contribute to better understanding of vestibular and oculomotor dysfunctions in HD, the latter being one of the main clinical features of HD.

Vonsattel et al. [11] reported on the basis of more than 1000 post-mortem brains that the cerebellum is only slightly smaller in grade 3 and 4 HD brains than in controls. He also detected that the mainly segmental loss of Purkinje cells is inconsistent across the HD brains examined. In contrast, Rüb et al. [33] found Purkinje cell loss in the cerebellum and loss of neurons in the four cerebellar nuclei. In a recent study, significant Purkinje cell loss was correlated with motor impairments, whereas no loss was associated with a major mood-phenotype in HD [34]. Notably, cerebellar atrophy is particularly pronounced in juvenile-onset HD individuals accompanied with neuronal loss and gliosis [35].

White matter degeneration is most obvious in telencephalic areas including the corpus callosum and internal capsula (**Figure 1A**) indicating a severe affection of interhemispheric commissural connections and projection fiber tracts between cortical and noncortical brain regions. White matter alterations occur early in HD as supported by post-mortem [36] and magnetic resonance studies [37, 38]. Fiber tracts that are less in HD focus are also early affected. The fornix connecting the hippocampus with mammillary bodies displays a reduction of 34% already in prodromal cases and 41% in manifest HD [39]. This study also shows that white matter pathology is partly due to myelin breakdown and reduction of oligodendrocyte genes.

All in all, for many cortical and noncortical areas including white matter and fiber tracts, detailed information is still limited and needs more specific interdisciplinary investigations to provide a better understanding of the regional pathology and respective functional impairments. Of note, HD may also be related to other neurodegenerative diseases, for example Alzheimer (AD) and Parkinson disease that could influence regional degeneration [19]. However, the frequency of the coexistence of AD in HD is similar to AD in general population [11]. These aspects have to be considered when evaluating the neuropathology of HD, especially at older ages. Finally, the variation in neuronal degeneration among different HD patients also reflects the heterogeneity in functional impairments and pathogenesis.

3. Mutant Huntingtin aggregates

Misfolded proteins are common in many neurodegenerative diseases such as amyloid plaques or neurofibrillary tangles in Alzheimer and Lewy bodies in Parkinson disease. However, Alzheimer and Parkinson diseases comprise a group of disorders with similar symptoms, but may be caused by various reasons. HD is caused by a single gene; therefore, studies on HD-specific aggregates are particularly useful, as they are well comparable among different HD-affected brains. The CAG trinucleotide repeat in the *HTT* gene leads on translation to a polyglutamine stretch at the N-terminus of the protein Htt. Misfolded fragments of the protein are detected as aggregated forms differing in size, shape and composition within the cell nucleus, soma, cell processes or optionally also in the intercellular space. The pathogenesis of aggregates is still unclear and the interplay between neurodegeneration and aggregation far from being understood.

In HD brains, misfolded proteins were first described as so-called inclusion bodies by conventional electron microscopy [40]. They were detected in the nucleus of neurons as membrane-less round structures that could be distinguished due to lighter homogenous appearance from the surrounding caryoplasm. This observation must have been more of an incidental finding, as intranuclear inclusions are relatively rare in adult-onset human HD brains and extremely difficult to detect without immunohistochemical staining. Similar intranuclear structures with fibrillar and granular composition were also detected in the first transgenic HD animal model, the R6/2 mouse, as documented in **Figure 2**, by conventional transmission electron microscopy. R6/2 mice express exon 1 of the human HD gene with 115–150 CAG repeats, develop symptoms very early with some features reflecting juvenile-onset HD and exhibit a widespread distribution of intranuclear inclusions in all brain areas [41, 42]. Next, in human HD brains, the presence of mHtt aggregates was confirmed in nuclei and axons by light- and electronmicroscopic mHtt- and Ubiquitin-immunohistochemistry [43]. Generation of the EM48 antibody, which is specific to N-terminal fragments of mHtt [44], confirmed and extended the localization of mHtt aggregates/inclusions in neuronal cytoplasm, dendrites, axons and synapses [45]. Since then, the presence of aggregates and/or inclusions became the characteristic hallmark for histopathology in human HD brains and the increasing number of small and large animal models. From the morphological viewpoint, the terms for aggregates and inclusions are heterogenously used and therefore confusing. Common descriptions are aggregates in the neuropil and inclusions localized intranuclear. Considering the heterogenous size and form in human HD brains [43], it is difficult to distinguish one from another. In this chapter, we try to use both simultaneously, if possible.

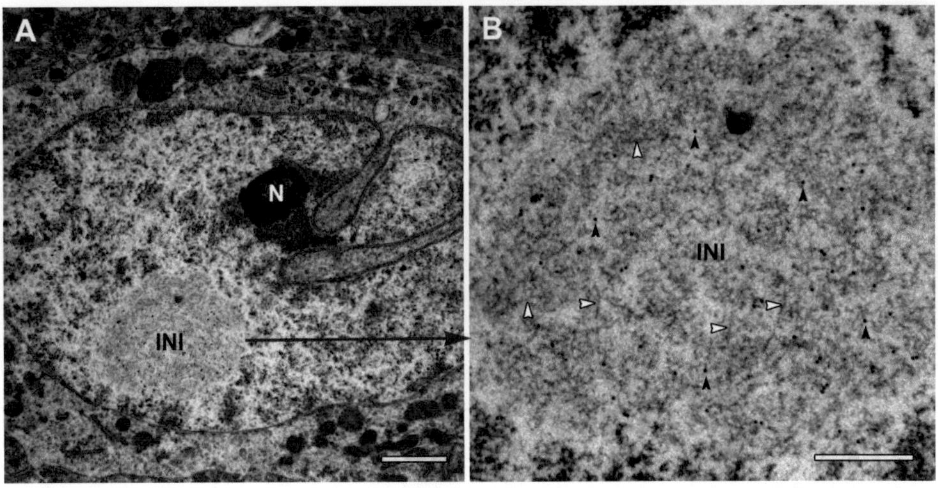

Figure 2.
Transmission electron microscopy of a cortical pyramidal neuron in R6/2 mouse. (A) The intranuclear inclusion (INI) is a membrane-less structure clearly distinguished from the surrounding chromatin in the caryoplasm and the nucleolus (N). (B) Enlargement of the INI reveals loosely arranged fibrillar (white arrowheads) and granular structures. Postembedding Ubiquitin immunogold staining exhibits particles (15 nm) localized in the INI (black arrowheads), not in caryoplasm. Bar in A = 1 µm; bar in B = 0.5 µm.

Studying mHtt aggregates/inclusions in the broad spectrum of HD animal models, it becomes apparent that the regional, cellular and subcellular localization is as diverse as the large number of HD models themselves. The use of different antibodies makes the assessment of comparable results still more difficult, furthermore, if strong retrievals are used prior to antibody incubation.

Nevertheless, it is undisputed that animal models are valuable to elucidate crucial aspects of underlying pathomechanisms, help to understand the neurological dysfunction and psychiatric alterations and are undispensable for the development of preclinical therapeutic approaches. The choice of an HD animal model will always depend on the underlying question. However, it has to be considered carefully to which extent the respective animal model could answer the respective question in human HD. To elucidate differences and similarities of mHtt aggregates, two established rodent models were presented here in more detail.

3.1 Aggregates in R6/2 mouse

The R6/2 mouse presents with behavioural and motor dysfunctions very early and shows severe other symptoms as progredient weight loss with affection of many peripheral organs leading to early death at 12–15 weeks of age [41]. According to their rapid and reproducible phenotype, they were early transferred to commercial breeding from where they are accessible by all interested scientists. The easy availability has also contributed to the fact that the R6/2 mouse has become one of the most extensively studied HD animal model.

Neuropathologically, the R6/2 mouse displays the greatest density of aggregates/inclusions, which makes this model extremely valuable when aggregates/inclusions are used for follow-up studies and/or *in vitro* and *in vivo* investigations of the misfolded proteins themselves. Therefore, the R6/2 mouse with abundant aggregates, the early and severe symptoms and a short life span has become a standard model for testing preclinical therapeutic approaches.

When investigating by conventional electron microscopy (**Figure 2**), intranuclear inclusions are easily detected in adult R6/2 mice in all brain areas inspected. As in human HD brains, the membrane-less intranuclear inclusion is clearly distinguished from the surrounding caryoplasm and comprises homogenously distributed fibrillar and granular structures (**Figure 2A** and **B**). Postembedding immunogold staining with Ubiquitin confirms intranuclear inclusion.

Immunostaining with EM48 antibody reveals an overall distribution of mHtt aggregates in all R6/2 brain areas. At cellular level, many neurons exhibit reactivity throughout the caryoplasm and a dense inclusion (**Figure 3A**). Immunoelectron microscopy confirmed nuclear distribution of EM48 reactivity loosely distributed in the caryoplasm and the dense intranuclear inclusion (**Figure 3B**). This observation extends the general assumption, that intranuclear mHtt is mainly localized as inclusion body. In R6/2 mice, the whole nucleus may harbour aggregates with varying expression. Nucleoli are always spared (**Figure 3B**). Of note, neurons with immunopositive caryoplasm show signs of degeneration as the irregular invaginated nuclear envelope starts to collapse indicating that mHtt may cause the cellular dysfunction finally leading to cell death (**Figure 3B**). The cytoplasm lacks mHtt reactivity. Single immunopositive spots were also detected in the surrounding neuropil. Taken together, the aggregates/inclusions in R6/2 mice are distributed across all brain areas, focussed on the caryoplasm and sparsely localized in the neuropil.

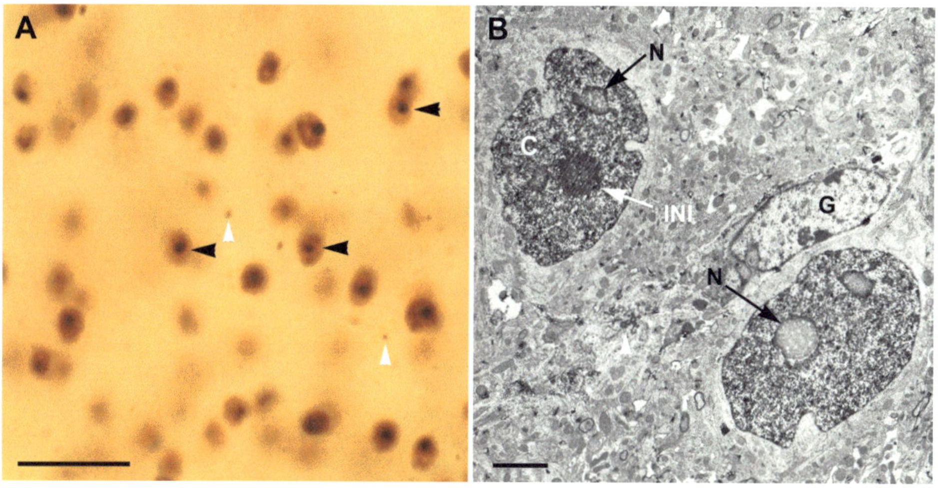

Figure 3.
EM48-immunohistochemistry in the striatum of R6/2 mouse. (A) Vibratome section (50 µm) displays brown-stained nuclei (black arrowheads) many of which with a black inclusion body. Single positive spots are distributed in the neuropil (white arrowheads). (B) Transmission immunoelectron microscopy confirms EM48 reactivity in the caryoplasm (C) densely arranged in the intranuclear inclusion (INI). Nucleoli (N) are spared. Immunopositive nuclei show irregular nuclear envelope. Adjacent glial cell nucleus (G) lacks EM48 reactivity. Bar in A = 100 µm; bar in B = 1 µm.

3.2 Aggregates in the tgHD rat

The transgenic rat model of HD (tgHD rat) carries a truncated htt cDNA fragment with 51 CAG repeats under control of the native rat promotor [46]. In contrast to the R6/2 mouse, the tgHD rat presents with slowly progressive motor and behavioural impairments reflecting the adult-onset phenotype of human HD individuals. Interestingly, the tgHD rat shares neuropathological similarities in regional distribution and subcellular composition of aggregates with human HD brains. In the tgHD rat und in human HD brain, aggregates are focussed on the ventral striatum and the extended amygdala [47–49] areas that are crucial for elucidating psychiatric aspects of the disease. In the tgHD rat, detailed transmission immunoelectron microscopy detected that aggregates are localized in medium-sized striatal neurons as small patches in neuronal cytoplasm, mitochondria, myelinated and unmylinated axons, synaptic terminals and, most frequently, loosely distributed or as large compact inclusions in dendrites and dendritic spines [48].

Aggregates are also localized in the nucleus (**Figure 4**). In contrast to the R6/2 mouse, the tgHD rat caryoplasm only exhibits very few small EM48-positive spots and occasionally a single inclusion (**Figure 4A** and **B**). Signs of degeneration are rarely observed in the striatal neurons. In sum, the tgHD rat shows a more regional mHtt distribution focussed on basal forebrain systems. On subcellular level, aggregates/inclusions may be detected in many parts of medium-sized striatal neurons.

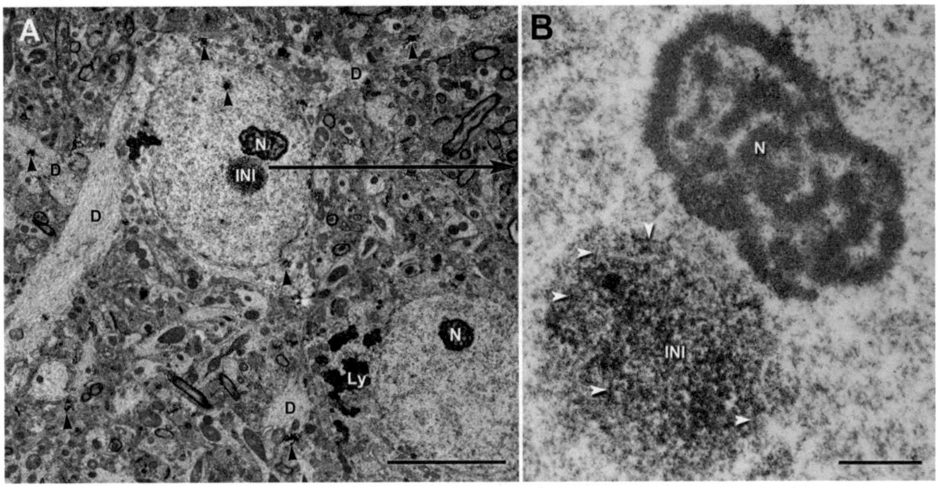

Figure 4.
EM48 immunohistochemistry in the neostriatum of tgHD rat. (A) Transmission electron microscopy shows an intranuclear inclusion (INI) in a normal appearing medium-sized neuron of a 23 months old tgHD rat. Some positive spots (black arrowheads) are also detected in the neuronal caryoplasm, cytoplasm and dendrites (D). (B) At higher enlargement the INI exhibits fibrillar (white arrowheads) and granular structures. Ly, lysosomes; bar in A = 5 μm; bar in B = 1 μm.

3.3 Aggregates in human HD brains

There are multiple studies on aggregates in HD animal models, but the localization of mHtt in human HD brains is less extensively investigated. In the studies of DiFiglia et al. and Gutekunst et al. [43, 45], important aspects of regional, cellular and subcellular aggregate localization were worked out in detail. Brains investigated included various Vonsattel grades as well as juvenile- and adult-onset HD brains. MHtt immunopositive intranuclear aggregates consistently called inclusion bodies by DiFiglia et al. [43] were more frequently detected in cortical layers of juvenile- than in adult-onset HD brains, in which they were predominantly detected in the neuropil in neuronal cell processes (called dystrophic neurites). The pronounced cortical localization in layers V and VI—especially in adult-onset HD individuals—was confirmed by Gutekunst et al. [45] for various cortical areas. Our investigations of selected frontal, parietal, temporal and occipital cortical areas by peroxidase EM48-immunohistochemistry also show that layers V and VI display the highest amount of aggregates/inclusions in varying degrees (unpublished results). The striatum, which is the first focus of studies in HD animal models, only displays a limited amount of aggregates in human HD brains, more expressed in the ventral than in the dorsal neostriatum [43, 45]. This observation was extended by our investigation, as we found aggregates/inclusions focussed to the accumbens and the extended amygdala [49], both functional-anatomical entities acting as interface between motor, limbic and olfactory-associated basal forebrain areas.

All human brains investigated in our cohort showed a heterogenous spectrum of aggregates differing in size, form and composition (**Figure 5A**). Confocal EM48 immunofluorescence counterstained with DAPI detected that most aggregates are localized in the neuropil, and only a few nuclei are associated with small positive spots (**Figure 5B**). Of note, it is relatively easy to localize aggregates in the nucleus and cytoplasm; however, the exact assignment to neuronal cell processes in the neuropil is difficult and awaits further detailed investigations using various techniques. One of the techniques to elucidate the fine structural composition of aggregates is transmission electron microscopy. Large inclusions often display an immunopositive rim with granular and vesicular structures and a mainly immunonegative core with densely arranged fibrillar structures (**Figure 5C**). In sum, in human HD brains aggregates/inclusions are predominantly localized in cortical areas, and—less expressed—in selected basal limbic-associated forebrain systems. Localization of aggregates/inclusions in many subcortical areas is less investigated and awaits further and more detailed investigation. Particularly, correlation studies between aggregate distribution and neurological dysfunctions are almost completely lacking in human HD.

A breakthrough to understand the mHtt structure at close to native cellular level was performed by the recently developed high-resolution cryo-electron tomography [50, 51]. This methods allows a three-dimensional imaging of cytosolic inclusions and aggregates [51]. Hela cells and mouse neurons transfected with GFP-tagged Htt exon 1 comprising 97 Q displayed inclusions which were identified by live cell imaging and further treated for cryo-electron tomography. Large mHtt inclusions are composed of organized centrally located fibrils, which interact with the membranes of the endoplasmic reticulum and deform their normal organization. This observation elucidates the subcellular machinery of mHtt aggregates and suggests a destructive effect of the inclusions. Comparing Bäuerlein's results with the large inclusions detected in the human HD brains investigated here by transmission electron microscopy (**Figure 5C**), it may look similar with the granular and vesicular structures in a more loosely arranged rim area and tightly packed fibrillar structures within the core. The question remains how far Bäuerlein's results reflect the broad spectrum of mHtt inclusions/aggregates in the human HD brain. Nevertheless provide these results important insights into cellular impairments by mHtt inclusions/aggregates and are encouraging findings, which show that the interdisciplinary research on subcellular level is currently on the way to complement one another.

For therapeutic approaches that target lowering of mHtt levels in the brain, it is of major interest to develop non-invasive tools as biomarkers to visualize mHtt during disease progression. Imaging agents visible by positron emission tomography would be extremely helpful to identify and track mHtt distribution prior and during the therapy. Recently, a high-affinity Fluorine-18 radioligand was developed for imaging mHtt aggregates in HD animal models and also human post-mortem HD brain tissue [52]. This PET-imaging agent showed sufficient brain uptake in rodents and

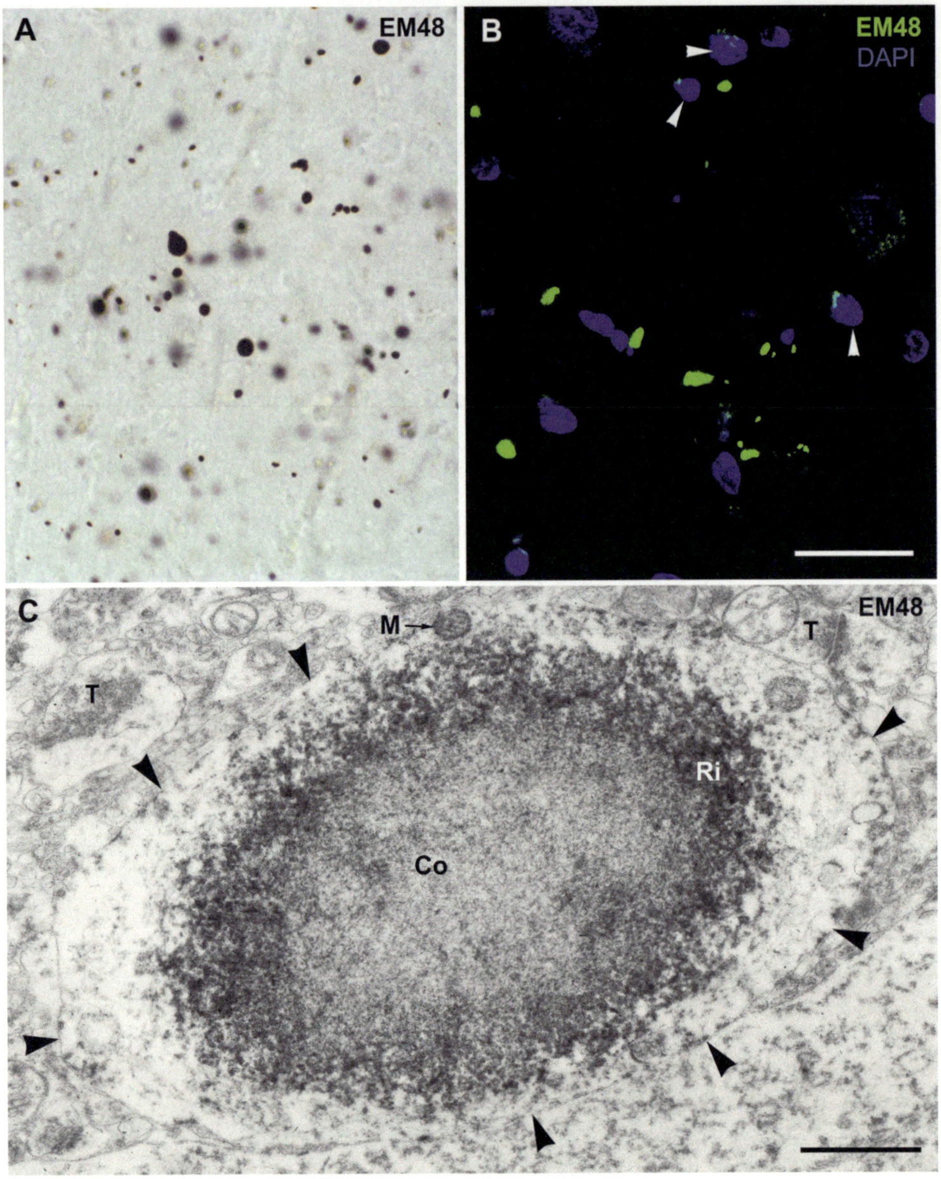

Figure 5.
EM48-immunohistochemistry in human HD brain (CAG 54/20). (A) Vibratome section (80 µm) displays distribution of mHtt aggregates varying in form and size localized in layer V and VI of the anterior cingulate cortex. (B) Confocal immunofluorescence of a cryosection (15 µm) with EM48 (green) counterstained with DAPI (blue) shows mainly neuropil aggregates. Some nuclei are associated with tiny positive dots (white arrowheads). (C) Transmission electron microscopy exhibits a large aggregate with an immunopositive rim (Ri) and a mainly immunonegative core (Co). Arrowheads mark the border of the neuropil structure harbouring the aggregate. M, mitochondrium; T, synaptic terminal; bar in B for A and B = 50 µm; bar in C = 1 µm.

non-human primates to be monitored *in vivo*. Furthermore, autogradiography with the ligand displayed specific binding on human post-mortem HD brain sections, which may correspond to aggregate accumulation as further indicated by mHtt-immunohistochemistry on adjacent sections. Even if such non-invasive studies are still at the very beginning, the application of radioligands as PET-imaging tracer in human HD brains to monitor alterations of mHtt localization would be of enormous benefit for controlling the course of therapy. It is also of crucial importance to carefully evaluate the validity of ligands as imaging biomarkers especially in mHtt-rich human brain areas, as localization of mHtt may be completely different from the before investigated animal model.

4. Conclusions

In HD, neurodegeneration is most expressed in striatal areas, but cortical and other noncortical areas are also severely affected including the grey and—especially in early HD—also the white matter. Notably, neurodegeneration is varying across the different HD brains, which may reflect the diversity in functional impairments of HD patients. For many brain areas, detailed information about macroscopic and microscopic affection is still limited and needs more specific interdisciplinary investigations to provide a better understanding of the regional neuropathology and related dysfunctions.

Aggregates/inclusions are the characteristic histopathological hallmark of HD. In HD animal models, the regional, cellular and subcellular localization is as diverse as the large number of models themselves with differently pronounced similarities to the human HD aggregation pattern. To date, the exact role of the Htt protein has not yet been clarified. The mechanism of formation and maturation of aggregates is currently intensively studied in living cell cultures providing first insights into the dynamic of mHtt and the toxic influence of aggregates and inclusion bodies. Furthermore, high-resolution techniques and improved tissue preservation are necessary to transfer the results on living cells to the aggregation process in human HD brains. So far, the controversial discussion about gain of function and toxicity in the interplay between aggregates and neurodegeneration is going on.

Acknowledgements

We are grateful to Anne Schlichting, Luzie Augostinowski, Katja Rumpf, Sabine Peuckert, Robert Nadgrabski, Claudia Schneider (Institute of Anatomy, Medical Faculty, Ruhr-University Bochum, Germany) for their excellent technical assistance.

The authorship criteria are listed in our Authorship Policy: https://www.intechopen.com/page/authorship-policy.

Conflict of interest

There are no conflicts of interest.

Author details

Elisabeth Petrasch-Parwez[1*], Hans-Werner Habbes[1], Marlen Löbbecke-Schumacher[1], Constanze Rana Parwez[2], Carsten Saft[3] and Sarah Maria von Hein[3]

1 Department of Neuroanatomy and Molecular Brain Research, Ruhr-University Bochum, Bochum, Germany

2 Department of Neurology, St. Josef's Hospital, Ruhr-University Bochum, Bochum, Germany

3 Department of Neurology, Huntington-Center NRW, St. Josef's Hospital, Ruhr-University Bochum, Bochum, Germany

*Address all correspondence to: elisabeth.petrasch-parwez@rub.de

References

[1] Macdonald M. A novel gene containing a trinucleotide repeat that is expanded and unstable on Huntington's disease chromosomes. Cell. 1993;**72**(6):971-983

[2] Langbehn D, Brinkman R, Falush D, Paulsen J, Hayden M, on behalf of an International Huntington's Disease Collaborative Group. A new model for prediction of the age of onset and penetrance for Huntington's disease based on CAG length: Prediction of the age of onset and penetrance for HD. Clinical Genetics. 2004;**65**(4): 267-277

[3] Andrew SE, Paul Goldberg Y, Kremer B, Telenius H, Theilmann J, Adam S, et al. The relationship between trinucleotide (CAG) repeat length and clinical features of Huntington's disease. Nature Genetics. 1993;**4**(4):398-403

[4] Quarrell O, O'Donovan KL, Bandmann O, Strong M. The prevalence of juvenile Huntington's disease: A review of the literature and meta-analysis. PLoS Current. 2012;**4**:e4f8606b742ef3

[5] Achenbach J, Thiels C, Lücke T, Saft C. Clinical manifestation of juvenile and pediatric HD patients: A retrospective case series. Brain Sciences. 2020;**10**(6):340

[6] Tabrizi SJ, Leavitt BR, Landwehrmeyer GB, Wild EJ, Saft C, Barker RA, et al. Targeting Huntingtin expression in patients with Huntington's disease. The New England Journal of Medicine. 2019;**380**(24):2307-2316

[7] Wild EJ, Tabrizi SJ. Therapies targeting DNA and RNA in Huntington's disease. The Lancet Neurology. 2017;**16**(10):837-847

[8] Meynert T. Discussion to Fritsch. Psychiatry. 1877;**4**:47

[9] Alzheimer A. Über die anatomische Grundlage der Huntingtonschen Chorea und der choreatischen Bewegungen überhaupt. Neurologisches Centralblatt. 1911;**30**:891-892

[10] Vonsattel J-P, Myers RH, Stevens TJ, Ferrante RJ, Bird ED, Richardson EP. Neuropathological classification of Huntington's disease. Journal of Neuropathology and Experimental Neurology. 1985;**44**(6):559-577

[11] Vonsattel JPG, Keller C, del Pilar Amaya M. Neuropathology of Huntington's disease. In: Handbook of Clinical Neurology [Internet]. Elsevier; 2008. pp. 599-618

[12] Myers RH, Vonsattel JP, Paskevich PA, Kiely DK, Stevens TJ, Cupples LA, et al. Decreased neuronal and increased oligodendroglial densities in Huntington's disease caudate nucleus. Journal of Neuropathology and Experimental Neurology. 1991; **50**(6):729-742

[13] Gómez-Tortosa E, MacDonald ME, Friend JC, Taylor SA, Weiler LJ, Cupples LA, et al. Quantitative neuropathological changes in presymptomatic Huntington's disease. Annals of Neurology. 2001;**49**(1): 29-34

[14] Sapp E, Kegel KB, Aronin N, Hashikawa T, Uchiyama Y, Tohyama K, et al. Early and progressive accumulation of reactive microglia in the Huntington disease brain. Journal of Neuropathology and Experimental Neurology. 2001;**60**(2):161-172

[15] Zuccato C, Ciammola A, Rigamonti D, Leavitt BR, Goffredo D, Conti L, et al.

Loss of Huntingtin-mediated BDNF gene transcription in Huntington's disease. Science. 2001;**293**(5529):493-498

[16] Clabough EBD. Huntington's disease: The past, present, and future search for disease modifiers. The Yale Journal of Biology and Medicine. 2013;**86**(2):217-233

[17] Ferrante RJ, Gutekunst C-A, Persichetti F, McNeil SM, Kowall NW, GusellaJF,etal.Heterogeneoustopographic and cellular distribution of Huntingtin expression in the normal human neostriatum. The Journal of Neuroscience. 1997;**17**(9):3052-3063

[18] Waldvogel HJ, Kim EH, Tippett LJ, Vonsattel JPG, Faull RL. The neuropathology of Huntington's disease. In: Nguyen HHP, Cenci MA, editors. Behavioral Neurobiology of Huntington's Disease and Parkinson's Disease [Internet]. Berlin, Heidelberg: Springer Berlin Heidelberg; 2014. pp. 33-80

[19] Hadzi TC, Hendricks AE, Latourelle JC, Lunetta KL, Cupples LA, Gillis T, et al. Assessment of cortical and striatal involvement in 523 Huntington disease brains. Neurology. 2012;**79**(16):1708-1715

[20] Lange H, Thörner G, Hopf A, Schröder KF. Morphometric studies of the neuropathological changes in choreatic diseases. Journal of the Neurological Sciences. 1976;**28**(4):401-425

[21] Singh-Bains MK, Waldvogel HJ, Faull RLM. The role of the human globus pallidus in Huntington's disease: Globus pallidus in HD. Brain Pathology. 2016;**26**(6):741-751

[22] Lange HW, Aulich A. Die Hirnatrophie bei der Huntingtonschen Krankheit. Stuttgart: Die Huntingtonsche Krankheit Hippokrates; 1986. pp. 25-41

[23] Rosas HD, Koroshetz WJ, Chen YI, Skeuse C, Vangel M, Cudkowicz ME, et al. Evidence for more widespread cerebral pathology in early HD: An MRI-based morphometric analysis. Neurology. 2003;**60**(10):1615-1620

[24] Johnson EB, Ziegler G, Penny W, Rees G, Tabrizi SJ, Scahill RI, et al. Dynamics of cortical degeneration over a decade in Huntington's disease. Biological Psychiatry. 2021;**89**(8):807-816

[25] Nana AL, Kim EH, Thu DCV, Oorschot DE, Tippett LJ, Hogg VM, et al. Widespread heterogeneous neuronal loss across the cerebral cortex in Huntington's disease. Journal of Huntingtons Diseases. 2014;**3**(1):45-64

[26] Thu DCV, Oorschot DE, Tippett LJ, Nana AL, Hogg VM, Synek BJ, et al. Cell loss in the motor and cingulate cortex correlates with symptomatology in Huntington's disease. Brain. 2010;**1339**(4):1094-1110

[27] Kassubek J, Juengling FD, Ecker D, Landwehrmeyer GB. Thalamic atrophy in Huntington's disease co-varies with cognitive performance: A morphometric MRI analysis. Cerebral Cortex. 2005;**15**(6):846-853

[28] Heinsen H, Rüb U, Gangnus D, Jungkunz G, Bauer M, Ulmar G, et al. Nerve cell loss in the thalamic centromedian-parafascicular complex in patients with Huntington's disease. Acta Neuropathologica. 1996;**91**(2): 161-168

[29] Heinsen H, Rüb U, Bauer M, Ulmar G, Bethke B, Schüler M, et al. Nerve cell loss in the thalamic mediodorsal nucleus in Huntington's disease. Acta Neuropathologica. 1999;**97**(6):613-622

[30] Soneson C, Fontes M, Zhou Y, Denisov V, Paulsen JS, Kirik D, et al. Early changes in the hypothalamic region in prodromal Huntington disease revealed by MRI analysis. Neurobiology of Disease. 2010;**40**(3):531-543

[31] van Wamelen DJ, Aziz NA. Hypothalamic pathology in Huntington disease. In: Handbook of Clinical Neurology [Internet]. Elsevier; 2021. pp. 245-255

[32] Rüb U, Hentschel M, Stratmann K, Brunt E, Heinsen H, Seidel K, et al. Huntington's disease (HD): Degeneration of select nuclei, widespread occurrence of neuronal nuclear and axonal inclusions in the brainstem: The brainstem in Huntington's disease. Brain Pathology. 2014;**24**(3):247-260

[33] Rüb U, Hoche F, Brunt ER, Heinsen H, Seidel K, Del Turco D, et al. Degeneration of the cerebellum in Huntington's disease (HD): Possible relevance for the clinical picture and potential gateway to pathological mechanisms of the disease process: The cerebellum in Huntington's disease. Brain Pathology. 2013;**23**(2):165-177

[34] Singh-Bains MK, Mehrabi NF, Sehji T, Austria MDR, Tan AYS, Tippett LJ, et al. Cerebellar degeneration correlates with motor symptoms in Huntington disease. Annals of Neurology. 2019;**85**(3):396-405

[35] Latimer CS, Flanagan ME, Cimino PJ, Jayadev S, Davis M, Hoffer ZS, et al. Neuropathological comparison of adult onset and juvenile Huntington's disease with cerebellar atrophy: A report of a father and son. Journal of Huntingtons Diseases. 2017;**6**(4):3377-3348

[36] Lange HW. Quantitative changes of telencephalon, diencephalon, and mesencephalon in Huntington's chorea, postencephalitic, and idiopathic parkinsonism. Verhandlungen der Anatomischen Gesellschaft. 1981;**75**:923-925

[37] Crawford HE, Hobbs NZ, Keogh R, Langbehn DR, Frost C, Johnson H, et al. Corpus callosal atrophy in premanifest and early Huntington's disease. Journal of Huntingtons Diseases. 2013;**2**(4):517-526

[38] Tabrizi SJ, Scahill RI, Owen G, Durr A, Leavitt BR, Roos RA, et al. Predictors of phenotypic progression and disease onset in premanifest and early-stage Huntington's disease in the TRACK-HD study: Analysis of 36-month observational data. The Lancet Neurology. 2013;**12**(7):637-649

[39] Gabery S, Kwa JE, Cheong RY, Baldo B, Ferrari Bardile C, Tan B, et al. Early white matter pathology in the fornix of the limbic system in Huntington disease. Acta Neuropathologica. 2021;**142**(5):791-806

[40] Roizin L, Stellar S, Willson N, Whittier J, Liu JC. Electron microscope and enzyme studies in cerebral biopsies of Huntington's chorea. Transactions of the American Neurological Association. 1974;**99**:240-243

[41] Mangiarini L, Sathasivam K, Seller M, Cozens B, Harper A, Hetherington C, et al. Exon 1 of the HD gene with an expanded CAG repeat is sufficient to cause a progressive neurological phenotype in transgenic mice. Cell. 1996;**87**(3):493-506

[42] Davies SW, Turmaine M, Cozens BA, DiFiglia M, Sharp AH, Ross CA, et al. Formation of neuronal intranuclear inclusions underlies the neurological dysfunction in mice transgenic for the HD mutation. Cell. 1997;**90**(3):537-548

[43] DiFiglia M, Sapp E, Chase KO, Davies SW, Bates GP, Vonsattel JP,

et al. Aggregation of Huntingtin in neuronal intranuclear inclusions and dystrophic neurites in brain. Science. 1997;**277**(5334):1990-1993

[44] Li H, Li S-H, Yu Z-X, Shelbourne P, Li X-J. Huntingtin aggregate-associated axonal degeneration is an early pathological event in Huntington's disease mice. The Journal of Neuroscience. 2001;**21**(21):8473-8481

[45] Gutekunst C-A, Li S-H, Yi H, Mulroy JS, Kuemmerle S, Jones R, et al. Nuclear and neuropil aggregates in Huntington's disease: Relationship to neuropathology. The Journal of Neuroscience. 1999;**19**(7):2522-2534

[46] von Horsten S, Schmitt I, Nguyen HP, Holzmann C, Schmidt T, Walther T, et al. Transgenic rat model of Huntington's disease. Human Molecular Genetics. 2003;**12**(6):617-624

[47] Nguyen HP, Kobbe P, Rahne H, Wörpel T, Jäger B, Stephan M, et al. Behavioral abnormalities precede neuropathological markers in rats transgenic for Huntington's disease. Human Molecular Genetics. 2006;**15**(21):3177-3194

[48] Petrasch-Parwez E, Nguyen H-P, Löbbecke-Schumacher M, Habbes H-W, Wieczorek S, Riess O, et al. Cellular and subcellular localization of Huntington aggregates in the brain of a rat transgenic for Huntington disease. The Journal of Comparative Neurology. 2007;**501**(5):716-730

[49] Petrasch-Parwez E, Habbes H-W, Lobbecke-Schumacher M, Saft C, Niescery J. The ventral striatopallidum and extended Amygdala in Huntington disease. In: Ferry B, editor. The Amygdala: A Discrete Multitasking Manager [Internet]. InTech; 2012

[50] Bäuerlein FJB, Saha I, Mishra A, Kalemanov M, Martínez-Sánchez A, Klein R, et al. In situ architecture and cellular interactions of PolyQ inclusions. Cell. 2017;**171**(1):179-187

[51] Bäuerlein FJB, Fernández-Busnadiego R, Baumeister W. Investigating the structure of neurotoxic protein aggregates inside cells. Trends in Cell Biology. 2020;**30**(12):951-966

[52] Kaur T, Brooks AF, Lapsys A, Desmond TJ, Stauff J, Arteaga J, et al. Synthesis and evaluation of a fluorine-18 radioligand for imaging Huntingtin aggregates by positron emission tomographic imaging. Frontiers in Neuroscience. 2021;**15**:766176

Chapter 2

Neuropathology of Huntington's Disease

Taylor G. Brown and Liam Chen

Abstract

Huntington's disease (HD) is a devastating neurodegenerative disease that results in motor, cognitive, and psychiatric impairments. HD results from an autosomal dominant polyglutamine expansion in the *huntingtin* (*HTT*) gene that results in a misfolded and aggregated protein. The disease is uniformly fatal and demonstrates characteristic neuropathological changes. While the striatum is preferentially affected, the cortex and many other brain regions are involved in pathogenesis and show progressive changes throughout the disease.

Keywords: Huntington, neuropathology, degeneration, striatum, aggregate

1. Introduction

This chapter summarizes the current knowledge of the neuropathological changes that occur in Huntington's disease (HD). HD is an autosomal dominant neurodegenerative disease caused by a polyglutamine expansion in the *huntingtin* gene [1]. The mutation was discovered in 1993 [1], however cases were first documented in 1872 by George Huntington [2]. The disease is characterized by progressive motor, cognitive, and psychiatric impairments and is uniformly fatal [3–6]. Analysis of postmortem brains reveals global atrophy of approximately 19–30% with 29–64% and 23–29% reductions in basal ganglia and cortical volume, respectively [7–9]. HD is thought to preferentially affect medium spiny neurons (MSNs) of the striatum and lead to their degeneration, however the exact reasons why MSNs are so vulnerable is still unknown [7, 10–12]. In addition to the striatum, HD affects other brain areas and peripheral tissues as well, though many of these areas are comparatively less studied.

2. Biological basis and symptomatology of HD

2.1 Biological basis of HD

HD is caused by a polyglutamine (CAG) expansion in exon 1 of the *huntingtin* gene (*HTT*). Normal individuals have stable repeat lengths up to 26, whereas repeat lengths from 27 to 35 are potentially unstable. HD is associated with CAG repeats of

IntechOpen

40 or more, with repeat lengths of 36–39 demonstrating incomplete penetrance [13]. The expanded CAG repeat produces a dysfunctional, unfolded, and aggregated huntingtin (HTT) protein, called mutant HTT (mHTT) [1]. The normal function of HTT is poorly understood, although some broad functions, such as roles in development, cell adhesion, and brain-derived neurotrophic factor transport and production, have been reported [14–16]. Not only does the expansion disrupt normal HTT functions, but it also exhibits toxic gain-of-function [16, 17]. While HTT is expressed in many cell types, medium spiny neurons (MSNs) of the striatum are particularly vulnerable to mHTT. While the exact mechanisms are still unclear, mHTT causes MSN death and leads to degeneration of the striatum [7, 11, 12].

2.2 HD symptomatology

HD causes motor, cognitive, and psychiatric deficits and the disease is uniformly fatal within a median time from motor symptom onset to death of 18 years [18]. The symptoms are severe and patients often lose independence rapidly, requiring constant care approximately 10 years after motor symptom onset [4]. The motor symptoms come in two broad categories: involuntary movements and impaired voluntary movement [3]. Involuntary movements such as chorea are common in the early stages of HD whereas the impaired voluntary movements, including coordination difficulties and bradykinesia, are often seen in later stages of the disease [4]. In addition, patients also have oculomotor abnormalities and dysdiadochokinesis among other motor symptoms [4]. Patients also experience cognitive symptoms, including personality changes, problems with attention and emotion recognition, cognitive slowing, initiation difficulties, and lack of awareness of deficits [4, 6]. Psychiatric symptoms include depressed mood, anxiety, apathy, irritability, social disengagement, and impulsivity [4, 5].

3. Basal ganglia

3.1 Normal basal ganglia

The basal ganglia is a set of subcortical nuclei located at the base of the forebrain [19]. This region is highly affected in HD [8] and thus, a review on its components, architecture, and circuitry is provided for context.

The basal ganglia is comprised of the striatum, globus pallidus (GP), subthalamic nucleus (STN), and substantia nigra (SN) [20]. The globus pallidus has two components, the internal and external segments (GPi and GPe respectively). The substantia nigra has two components, the pars reticulata (SNr) and the pars compacta (SNc) [19, 20].

The striatum gets input from many cortical areas, integrates the information, and sends it in multiple pathways throughout the basal ganglia [21]. The two major pathways are the direct and indirect pathways. The direct pathway is a monosynaptic pathway from the striatum to the GPi, whereas the indirect pathway is multisynaptic. The indirect pathway has projections from the striatum to the GPe, the GPe to the STN, and the STN to the GPi [19, 22–24]. The two pathways converge at GPi and send inhibitory projections to the ventral anterior and ventral lateral nuclei of the thalamus. Disruption or imbalance of these pathways can lead to motor dysfunction [25].

3.1.1 Striatum

The dorsal striatum is comprised of the caudate and the putamen, while the ventral striatum is nucleus accumbens. Running between the caudate and the putamen is the internal capsule [26].

The striatum itself is a heterogenous region with two compartments—the matrix and the striosomes. The compartments differ based on their efferent and afferent connections as well as their neurochemical makeup. The striosomes receive inputs from the SNc, prefrontal cortex, and limbic system and they send outputs to the SNc [27]. The matrix compartment receives inputs from motor, somatosensory, frontal, parietal, and occipital cortices and the matrix sends outputs to GPe, GPi, and SNr [27]. The matrix strongly expresses acetylcholinesterase (AChE) whereas the striosomes only weakly stains for AChE [28]. Additionally, there are many other markers that can differentiate between striosome or matrix compartments, such as tyrosine hydroxylase or enkephalin [29].

The striatum contains multiple types of neurons and glial cells [3]. MSNs are GABAergic projection neurons that make up 90–95% of the striatal neuronal population [3, 30]. They receive glutamatergic input from many brain areas including the cortex and some thalamic nuclei [31–33] as well as dopaminergic input from the SN [27, 30]. MSNs that are in the direct pathway and project to the GPi express dopamine D1 receptors while MSNs in the indirect pathway express D2 receptors [22, 30]. Besides MSNs, the striatum also contains several classes of interneurons, the most abundant of which are large cholinergic interneurons [30, 34].

3.2 HD striatum

The dorsal striatum shows significant bilateral atrophy with striking caudate and putamen volume loss (**Figure 1A**) [7]. The degeneration typically occurs from the tail of the caudate to the head and body (caudal to rostral, dorsal to ventral, and medial to lateral) [36]. The particular sequence of degeneration is described further in Section 8.

Within the striatum, MSNs experience profound degeneration (**Figure 1B** and **C**) [3]. In general striatal interneurons are not very affected in HD [3, 37, 38], with the exception of parvalbumin-containing interneurons which degenerate significantly and in a grade-dependent manner [39]. Some cases of HD show rare but distinct, round striatal areas of preservation called islets. They measure 0.5–1.0 mm and show normal neuronal density but increased astrocyte density [40, 41].

Nearly all evidence suggests that cells displaying the classic apoptotic morphology are extremely rare in HD [42]. Remaining MSNs in HD brains appear to be smaller but maintain their normal somatic morphology [36]. Degenerating neurons, called "neostriatal dark neurons" appear darker than healthy neurons and have scalloped cellular membranes, granular dark cytoplasm, and condensed chromatin [29]. These dark neurons are typically present between atrophic and normal areas of the striatum [36]. Besides these atrophic neurons, ballooned neurons are extremely common in affected regions of HD brains. These neurons have enlarged, basophilic cytoplasm with flattened nuclei and Nissl substance and lipofuscin granules at the nuclear periphery [26, 43].

3.2.1 Matrix and striosome

The heterogenous, patchy nature of mHTT reactivity in the striatum of HD patients was observed and determined to reflect the distribution of striatal

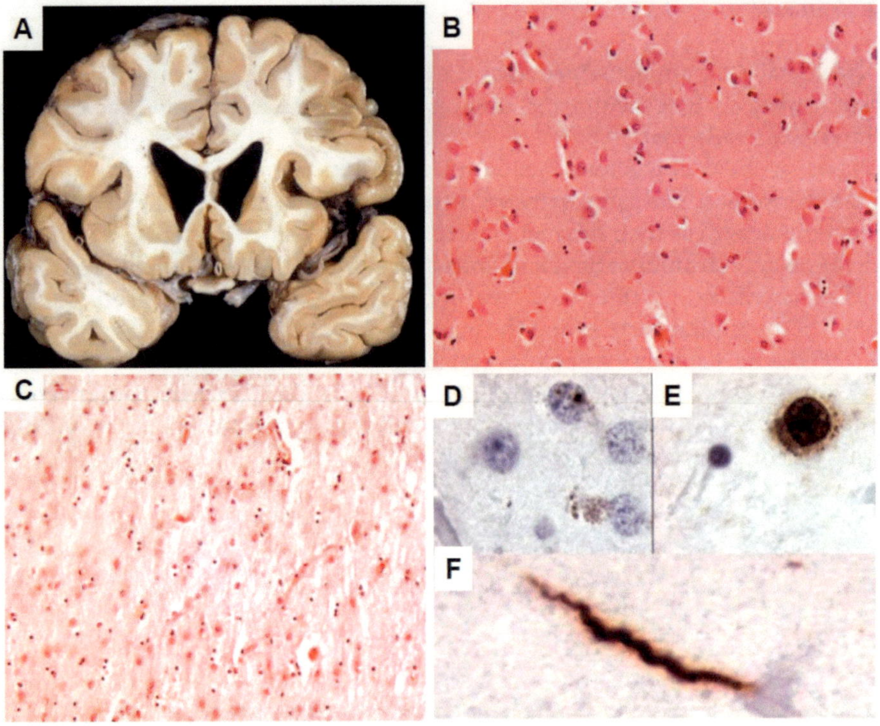

Figure 1.
Neuropathology of HD. (A) Coronal section of fixed brain at the level of the nucleus accumbens. Note HD grade 4 severe atrophy of the striatum and marked enlargement of the lateral ventricles. Normal (B) and grade 3 HD (C) putamen. Note severe neuron loss and astrocytosis. Immunohistochemical staining with 1C2 antibody against expanded polyglutamine of the TATA binding protein [35] demonstrates intranuclear inclusions, cytoplasmic granules (D and E) and neuritic aggregates (F) in cerebral cortex.

compartments. In early studies of HD, HTT was predominantly found in the matrix [44]. Many reports focusing on neurodegeneration found either matrix [45, 46] or striosome [47, 48] predominance, and in particular, discrepancies between compartments were evident in early disease stages. Further investigation into this phenomenon revealed that matrix or striosome predominance correlated with symptom type, where HD patients who showed preferential neuronal loss in striosomes tended to experience more mood dysfunction and HD patients who showed preferential matrix neuronal loss showed mainly motor symptoms [49]. It should be noted that many brains do not show any matrix or striosome predominance, so this phenomenon seems to be ungeneralizable, and it is possible for either compartment to experience predominant neuronal loss.

3.2.2 Indirect and direct pathway

While some studies have shown no differences between indirect and direct pathway MSN degeneration [50], other studies have shown that indirect, D2 receptor-positive MSNs degenerate and show dysfunction prior to direct, D1 receptor-positive MSNs [10, 51–53]. This predominant neuronal loss of indirect pathway MSNs occurs early and by late disease stages, no difference between pathways is noted [51, 52].

3.3 HD globus pallidus, STN, SN

The GP shows atrophy in grades 3 and 4, with more significant atrophy of the GPe than the GPi [36, 40, 43]. GP volume is decreased significantly [54, 55], but the density of neurons is maintained, suggesting minimal neuronal degeneration [36, 40]. Reactive gliosis is seen in the GPe in late stages of the disease [36].

The STN shows marked atrophy in grades 3 and 4, but no reactive astrocytes are seen in this region [36, 54]. An approximately 20% reduction in STN neuron number are seen in HD brains compared to control brains [56].

The SN pathology differs by component [36]. There is a loss of neurons in the SNr, whereas the SNc is more controversial, appearing thin but with an unchanged number of neurons in some studies [57, 58]. Other studies, however, claim to see a reduction of neuron number in the SNc, although to a lesser degree than in the SNr [59, 60].

3.4 Physiological and neurochemical changes

The loss of MSNs likely causes reductions in NMDA, GABA, and cannabinoid receptor binding in the striatum of HD patients [49, 61–63]. In the GPe, enkephalin staining is diminished as enkephalin-containing MSNs projecting to the GPe are lost and in the GPi and SNr, substance P staining is diminished as substance P-containing MSNs are lost [10, 51, 52, 64]. In addition, urea levels in the brains of HD patients are elevated, even at early disease stages, which suggests disrupted urea metabolism may play a role in neurodegeneration or neurological impairment in HD [65]. Vitamin B5, the precursor for coenzyme A, is reduced in HD patient brains and may contribute to neurodegeneration, as genetic defects in the coenzyme A biosynthetic pathway lead to neurodegeneration [66, 67].

It is thought that excitoxicity and synaptic changes may play a role in cell death. Many studies using animal models of HD have shown a variety of factors, such as astrocyte dysfunction, defects in energy metabolism, or altered cortical input, that could contribute to the MSN vulnerability to excitotoxity [68–73]. HD animal models also show early loss of corticostriatal and thalamostriatal synapses [74]. In postmortem brain tissue from HD patients, it was found that bassoon, an anchoring protein in the active zone, and HTT interact and this process draws bassoon into aggregates, causing a reduction of active zone proteins which may impair synaptic function [75].

4. Pathology in other brain regions

In addition to the basal ganglia, HD affects other brain regions such as the cortex, thalamus, cerebellum, brainstem nuclei, subventricular zone, hypothalamus, hippocampus, and white matter. In general, striatal pathology severity correlates well with pathology in other brain regions, though striatal pathology often precedes pathology elsewhere [36].

4.1 Cortex

Cortical pathology is a significant yet disputed component of HD [36]. Early reports on HD pathology either saw significant cortical atrophy [76] or minimal to absent cortical pathology [77]. Currently, the consensus suggests that there is indeed cortical atrophy, cortical thinning, and cortical volume loss [8, 9, 78]. Exactly which layer of cortical neurons is most affected is still under investigation, as some studies have reported involvement of layers V and VI [79, 80] and others have reported layers III and V [81]. Layers III and V project to the striatum so it has been hypothesized that pathology here could be retrograde from the striatum, however layer VI involvement questions this. It is fairly clear, however, that pyramidal neurons degenerate more than cortical interneurons [81, 82], though there may be heterogenous involvement of cortical interneurons and it may differ by HD patient [29].

Particular cortical regions, such as the motor cortex [82, 83], prefrontal cortex [80, 84], entorhinal cortex [79], cingulate cortex [83], and primary sensory areas [85], have been studied and each shows HD pathology, though it appears to vary between HD patients [86]. It is possible that degeneration and thinning of these particular areas may correlate with specific HD symptoms. One study showed that cases with significant motor cortex pathology showed profound motor dysfunction whereas cases with anterior cingulate cortex pathology showed predominance of mood symptoms [83, 87].

4.2 Cerebellum

Cerebellar involvement in HD is rather controversial. The cerebellum plays roles in motor coordination and control, attention, and many other processes [88–90]. Earliest reports of HD neuropathology did not note any cerebellar pathology [77], however recent studies have varied in their assessment of cerebellar atrophy, volume loss, and degeneration [3, 36, 91]. Vonsattel and others reported that the cerebellum displayed normal neuronal density but was atrophied in late stage HD brains [36, 92]. However, other studies were reporting the density of Purkinje cells were reduced by half [3]. A systematic study using serial sections of the cerebellum in HD brains showed widespread loss of Purkinje cells and degeneration of neurons in the deep cerebellar nuclei present at early stages of HD [91]. Interestingly, when HD patients are separated by symptom predominance, those with predominant motor symptoms had significant loss of Purkinje cells whereas those with predominant mood symptoms did not show any loss of Purkinje cells in the neocerebellum [93]. This cerebellar pathology is reminiscent of that seen in spinocerebellar ataxias (1, 2, and 3), and it is possible that HD has more similarities with these diseases than previously thought [94–96]. Classic cerebellar dysfunction signs such as gait abnormalities, dysarthria, oculomotor abnormalities, and fine motor skill impairment have indeed been reported in HD [3, 97–99].

4.3 Other brain areas

HD cases appear to show varied levels of thalamic pathology [100]. The thalamus often appears grossly normal but does show pathology in later stages, though this varies by thalamic nucleus [40]. The thalamus appears normal at early disease stages but at late disease stages, astrocytosis and neuronal loss are seen in the centromedial nucleus [36]. Atrophy has been reported in the centromedial/parafascicular nucleus, the dorsomedial nucleus, and the centromedial/ventrolateral nucleus group [100–102].

The hypothalamus is another area that shows HD pathology [55, 103, 104]. HD patients present with sleep disturbances, altered circadian rhythm, and weight loss

[105–107]. Atrophy, gliosis, and 90% cell loss of the lateral tuberal nucleus has been reported [3]. Other studies have shown a loss of orexin-positive and somatostatin-positive neurons in the lateral hypothalamus [108–110].

Early HD reports did not observe changes in hippocampal density [77], however more recent studies have found a 20% reduction of area [9], 9% reduction of volume [111], and neuronal loss and astrocytosis [36] in the hippocampus. It seems that changes in neuronal density may be restricted to the CA1 region [112].

The subventricular zone (SVZ), which is a region that contains adult stem cells and is located at the edge of the caudate nucleus, shows thickening that progresses with increasing grades of HD [113]. There was increased cell proliferation [113] and altered lipid architecture [114] in the SVZ of HD patients as well.

White matter changes occur in HD and the loss of white matter correlates with amount of gray matter lost [9]. Diffusion tensor imaging and MRI show presymptomatic white matter changes in the microstructure of the corpus callosum and internal capsule [115, 116].

Lastly, brainstem nuclei show pathology in HD. The brainstem shows widespread neuronal loss with particular involvement of the substantia nigra, precerebellar pontine nuclei, inferior olive, oculomotor reticulotegmental nucleus, premotor oculomotor area, raphe interpositus nucleus, auditory superior olive, and the vestibular nuclei [26, 117, 118]. HD patients present with autonomic disturbances and oculomotor dysfunction [4, 119], some of which could be explained by brainstem pathology.

5. Aggregates

Expanded HTT accumulates and forms aggregates and inclusions (**Figure 1D–F**) [120–122]. Normally, HTT is found mostly in the cytoplasm, dendrites, and axon terminals, but in HD, inclusions are also seen in the nucleus [123]. There are both intranuclear and extranuclear inclusions in HD [124] and they appear round or oblong, ranging from approximately 0.5–20 μm in diameter [123]. mHTT inclusions are found in neurons most commonly but also astrocytes, oligodendrocytes, and microglia [125, 126]. They are found more commonly in gray matter than white matter [123]. The aggregates can be detected prior to symptom onset [127].

A high density of aggregates are homogenously distributed throughout the striatum of HD brains [123]. No distinction between striosome and matrix compartments were noted in terms of aggregate load [123]. There is a high aggregate load in layers V and VI of the cortex as well [123]. Specifically, the insular and cingulate cortex had a high density of aggregates while other cortical areas and the SN, thalamus, hypothalamus, brainstem nuclei, GP, hippocampus, and cerebellum showed a much lower density [123]. Interestingly, mHTT aggregates are also found in the olfactory bulb of HD patients, though aggregate load here does not correlate with Vonsattel grading score [128].

Polyglutamine proteins can be detected using antibodies that recognize polyglutamine stretches, such as IC2. IC2 is a monoclonal antibody that predominantly binds to pathologic repeat lengths and can therefore detect mHTT [35]. It has consistently been used to detect mHTT aggregates in postmortem HD brains [129, 130]. Other studies have used EM48, an antibody that detects the N-terminal region of HTT, to detect HTT aggregates [123].

6. Pathology in peripheral tissues

HTT is expressed in many tissues and organs outside of the brain [105]. Besides the classic neurological symptoms, HD patients exhibit weight loss, atrophy of skeletal muscle, cardiac dysfunction, testicular atrophy, impaired glucose tolerance, and osteoporosis [105]. While the symptoms have been documented in patients [105, 131, 132], most of the research in peripheral tissue pathology is in HD animal models.

Postmortem samples from HD patients showed testicular atrophy and spermatogenesis deficits, with fewer spermatocytes and spermatids. Additionally, thicker walls and cross-sectional area of the seminiferous tubules were noted. In their study, the patient with the longest repeat length had the most severe testicular pathology [133].

Skeletal muscle atrophy is another hallmark of HD [134]. Muscle cells express mHTT and show inclusion bodies in animal models of HD [135, 136] and in muscle cell cultures from HD patients [137]. In addition to aggregate formation, cultured cells from HD patients also show mitochondrial abnormalities [137–139], and the two may work together to cause muscle wasting in HD.

Cardiac failure is relatively common among HD patients, as it occurs in about 30% of cases [132]. Cardiac tissue expresses HTT and while mHTT inclusions are seen in HD mice [140], no aggregates have been reported in cardiac tissue from HD patients [136]. Altered autonomic input to the heart [141], calcium dysregulation [142], and conduction abnormalities [111] are all seen in HD patients and could contribute to heart conditions.

The exact mechanisms that cause peripheral pathology are not fully understood. It is likely that cells that express aggregates are affected cell-autonomously to at least some extent, but the contribution of brain-derived hormones, signals from affected brain areas, or the degeneration of autonomic nerves is still being uncovered.

7. Gliosis

Gliosis is a significant part of HD pathology [143]. Microglia, astrocytes, and oligodendrocytes all show changes in response to HD [7, 36, 144–146]. The density of oligodendrocytes increases in the striatum of HD brains [36] and is particularly evident in early disease stages [127, 144].

Reactive microglia are seen in the striatum, cortex, and globus pallidus of HD patients in all grades of pathology and their number correlates with the degree of neuronal loss in the striatum [145, 146]. Positron emission tomography scans indicate that progressive microglia activation is also seen in the anterior cingulate cortex and prefrontal cortex [147]. In fact, this microglia activation was even seen in presymptomatic HD patients [148].

In addition to microglia, astrocytes play an important role as well. Glial fibrillary acidic protein (GFAP)-positive astrocytes are a component of the Vonsattel grading system (below) [7]. GFAP-positive astrocytes have traditionally been viewed as the reactive type, although the complexity of astrocyte heterogeneity and reactivity is still being uncovered [143, 149–152]. GFAP-positive astrocyte number in the striatum increases progressively with disease severity and striatal neurodegeneration [7]. Despite cortical atrophy and pathology, no astrocytosis was noted in prefrontal cortex samples from HD patients [84, 143].

8. Grading

The Vonsattel grading system was developed in 1985 and utilizes both macroscopic and microscopic pathology in the striatum to categorize the severity of HD degeneration [7, 26, 36].

Grade 0—These brains show no gross abnormalities despite clinical evidence of HD. There may be up to 30–40% reduction in neuron number in the head of the caudate, though no reactive astrocytes are present at this stage.

Grade 1—Macroscopically, there is mild atrophy of the caudate tail and body. The head of the caudate and the putamen may still appear normal. Microscopically, the neuronal loss and astrocytosis is predominantly in the tail of the caudate nucleus with lesser involvement of the caudate body and head and the nearby putamen.

Grade 2—Macroscopically, some atrophy of the caudate is seen with resulting enlargement of the lateral ventricles, although the ventricular surface maintains its convex shape. Microscopically, significant neuronal loss and reactive astrocytosis is seen in the dorsal parts of the caudate and putamen. The globus pallidus begins to show degeneration, with the GPe degenerating before the GPi.

Grade 3—Macroscopically, there is significant atrophy of the caudate, causing the ventricular surface to appear straight as it now parallels the internal capsule boundary. Microscopically, the neuronal loss and reactive astrocytosis is visible throughout the caudate and putamen and becomes severe. This pathology progresses dorsal to ventral, rostral to caudal, and medial to lateral in the striatum. Mild pathology is present in the nucleus accumbens.

Grade 4—Macroscopically, there is severe atrophy of the striatum causing the ventricular surface to become concave. Microscopically, severe striatal neuron loss reaches approximately 95% and there is severe astrocytosis. The globus pallidus volume is reduced by half and the nucleus accumbens may begin to show more significant pathology.

9. Juvenile HD

Juvenile HD occurs when disease onset manifests before 20 years of age [4, 153, 154], 75% of juvenile HD patients have inherited the mutation from their father. Paternal inheritance is associated with increased likelihood of repeat-length expansion, leading to earlier onset in the next generation, referred to as "anticipation" [155]. It is difficult to diagnose because it often presents with minimal chorea. Instead, behavioral symptoms are more prominent than motor symptoms at such early ages [4] and the motor symptoms that do prevail are typically rigidity and bradykinesia [3]. Contrary to adult-onset HD, juvenile cases are prone to seizures as well [3, 153].

Juvenile HD patient brains typically show more severe striatal pathology than adult HD brains [3]. Magnetic resonance imaging (MRI), magnetic resonance spectroscopy, and postmortem brains of juvenile HD patients show severe and early striatal volume loss accompanied by reduced neuronal density but no significant cortical or white matter involvement [156]. Interestingly, juvenile cases of HD show more islets than adult cases [40]. In general, neuronal intranuclear inclusions are more common in juvenile than adult HD [123]. Aggregate load in the striatum is also more significant in juvenile HD brains [157].

Compared to adult onset HD, juvenile HD brains show severe cerebellar atrophy [36, 158]. In one case study involving a father with adult onset HD and a son with juvenile HD, significantly more cerebellar pathology, including mHTT inclusions in cerebellar neurons, was seen in the juvenile case than the adult case [155]. In addition to the cerebellum, the GPi, thalamus, and nucleus accumbens are also more severely affected in juvenile HD patients [157, 159]. The frontal and parietal regions show gross atrophy and MRI analysis showed more widespread and faster cortical volume loss in juvenile cases compared to adult onset cases [157, 160].

10. Developmental changes

While HD is being increasingly recognized as a developmental disease, few neuropathological studies of developing brains with adult onset HD exist. Using tissue from HD carrier fetuses, it was found that HTT is mislocalized in ventricular zone progenitor cells, which disrupts the neuroepithelial junctional complexes and interkinetic nuclear migration [161]. This causes progenitor cells to prematurely enter into lineage specification [161]. Using imaging approaches, it has been shown that there is an absence of Sylvian fissure asymmetry, which occurs early in development, in the brains of HD patients [162]. Early genetic testing has allowed for imaging studies in children well prior to HD onset. In children with expanded repeats as young as 6 years old, increased connectivity between the striatum and other brain regions is evident [163]. Additionally, imaging has shown that these children have larger striatal volumes early in life, but more rapid decline in volume through aging [164].

Developmental malformations are not uncommon in HD patients. A recent study using a large cohort of autopsy brains found that developmental malformations were found approximately 6 times more frequently in HD-brains than in non HD-brains, with heterotopias being the most common malformation, though other asymmetric and solitary malformations were also seen [165].

11. Conclusion

HD is a complex neurodegenerative disease that involves multiple brain areas. In fact, it has taken decades to firmly establish that HD is not only a basal ganglia disorder, but rather affects many regions in a symptomatically relevant manner. Therefore, the neuropathology of HD is constantly being re-evaluated and studied. It is clear, however, that this disease causes significant striatal atrophy and neuronal loss with concomitant cortical changes that result in devastating motor, cognitive, and psychiatric consequences for HD patients.

Conflict of interest

The authors declare no conflict of interest.

Author details

Taylor G. Brown and Liam Chen*
University of Minnesota, Minneapolis, USA

*Address all correspondence to: llchen@umn.edu

References

[1] The Huntington's Disease Collaborative Research Group. A novel gene containing a trinucleotide repeat that is expanded and unstable on Huntington's disease chromosomes. Cell. 1993;**72**:971-983

[2] Huntington G. On chorea. Medical and Surgical Reporter. 1872;**26**:317-321

[3] Kremer B, Weber B, Hayden MR. New insights into the clinical features, pathogenesis and molecular genetics of Huntington disease. Brain Pathology (Zurich, Switzerland). 1992;**2**:321-335

[4] Bates GP, Dorsey R, Gusella JF, Hayden MR, Kay C, Leavitt BR, et al. Huntington disease. Nature Reviews Disease Primers. 2015;**1**:15005

[5] Paoli RA, Botturi A, Ciammola A, Silani V, Prunas C, Lucchiari C, et al. Neuropsychiatric burden in Huntington's disease. Brain Sciences. 2017;**7**:67

[6] Paulsen JS. Cognitive impairment in Huntington disease: Diagnosis and treatment. Current Neurology and Neuroscience Reports. 2011;**11**: 474-483

[7] Vonsattel J-P, Myers RH, Stevens TJ, Ferrante RJ, Bird ED, Richardson EP Jr. Neuropathological classification of Huntington's disease. Journal of Neuropathology and Experimental Neurology. 1985;**44**:559-577

[8] Halliday GM, McRitchie DA, Macdonald V, Double KL, Trent RJ, McCusker E. Regional specificity of brain atrophy in Huntington's disease. Experimental Neurology. 1998;**154**:663-672

[9] de la Monte SM, Vonsattel J-P, Richardson EP Jr. Morphometric demonstration of atrophic changes in the cerebral cortex, White matter, and Neostriatum in Huntington's disease. Journal of Neuropathology and Experimental Neurology. 1988;**47**:516-525

[10] Albin RL, Reiner A, Anderson KD, Dure LS, Handelin B, Balfour R, et al. Preferential loss of striato-external pallidal projection neurons in presymptomatic Huntington's disease. Annals of Neurology. 1992;**31**:425-430

[11] Ehrlich ME. Huntington's disease and the striatal medium spiny neuron: Cell-autonomous and non-cell-autonomous mechanisms of disease. Neurotherapeutics: The Journal of the American Society for Experimental NeuroTherapeutics. 2012;**9**:270-284

[12] Morigaki R, Goto S. Striatal vulnerability in Huntington's disease: Neuroprotection versus neurotoxicity. Brain Sciences. 2017;**7**:63

[13] Rubinsztein DC, Leggo J, Coles R, Almqvist E, Biancalana V, Cassiman J-J, et al. Phenotypic characterization of individuals with 30-40 CAG repeats in the Huntington disease (HD) gene reveals HD cases with 36 repeats and apparently Normal elderly individuals with 36-39 repeats. American Journal of Human Genetics. 1996;**59**:16-22

[14] Tousley A, Iuliano M, Weisman E, Sapp E, Richardson H, Vodicka P, et al. Huntingtin associates with the actin cytoskeleton and α-actinin isoforms to influence stimulus dependent morphology changes. PLoS One. 2019;**14**:e0212337

[15] Zeitlin S, Liu J-P, Chapman DL, Papaioannou VE, Efstratiadis A. Increased apoptosis and early embryonic lethality in mice nullizygous for the Huntington's disease gene homologue. Nature Genetics. 1995;**11**:155-163

[16] Schulte J, Littleton JT. The biological function of the huntingtin protein and its relevance to Huntington's disease pathology. Current Trends in Neurology. 2011;**5**:65-78

[17] Saudou F, Humbert S. The biology of huntingtin. Neuron. 2016;**89**:910-926

[18] Ross CA, Aylward EH, Wild EJ, Langbehn DR, Long JD, Warner JH, et al. Huntington disease: Natural history, biomarkers and prospects for therapeutics. Nature Reviews. Neurology. 2014;**10**:204-216

[19] Nambu A. Basal ganglia: Physiological circuits. In: Squire LR, editor. Encycl Neurosci [Internet]. Oxford: Academic Press; 2009. pp. 111-117. Available from: https://www.sciencedirect.com/science/article/pii/B9780080450469012985

[20] Nauta WJ, Domesick VB. Afferent and efferent relationships of the basal ganglia. Ciba Foundation Symposium. 1984;**107**:3-29

[21] Graybiel AM. The basal ganglia. Trends in Neurosciences. 1995;**18**:60-62

[22] Smith Y, Bevan MD, Shink E, Bolam JP. Microcircuitry of the direct and indirect pathways of the basal ganglia. Neuroscience. 1998;**86**:353-387

[23] Alexander GE, Crutcher MD. Functional architecture of basal ganglia circuits: Neural substrates of parallel processing. Trends in Neurosciences. 1990;**13**:266-271

[24] Albin RL, Young AB, Penney JB. The functional anatomy of basal ganglia disorders. Trends in Neurosciences. 1989;**12**:366-375

[25] DeLong MR. Primate models of movement disorders of basal ganglia origin. Trends in Neurosciences. 1990;**13**:281-285

[26] Rüb U, Seidel K, Heinsen H, Vonsattel JP, den Dunnen WF, Korf HW. Huntington's disease (HD): The neuropathology of a multisystem neurodegenerative disorder of the human brain. Brain Pathology. 2016;**26**:726-740

[27] Gerfen CR, Herkenham M, Thibault J. The neostriatal mosaic: II. Patch- and matrix-directed mesostriatal dopaminergic and non-dopaminergic systems. Journal of Neuroscience is an Official Journal of the Society for Neuroscience. 1987;**7**:3915-3934

[28] Graybiel AM, Ragsdale CW. Histochemically distinct compartments in the striatum of human, monkeys, and cat demonstrated by acetylthiocholinesterase staining. Proceedings of the National Academy of Sciences of the United States of America. 1978;**75**:5723-5726

[29] Waldvogel HJ, Kim EH, Tippett LJ, Vonsattel J-PG, Faull RLM. The neuropathology of Huntington's disease. Current Topics in Behavioral Neurosciences. 2015;**22**:33-80

[30] Lanciego JL, Luquin N, Obeso JA. Functional neuroanatomy of the basal ganglia. Cold Spring Harbor Perspectives in Medicine. 2012;**2**:a009621

[31] Carpenter MB, Nakano K, Kim R. Nigrothalamic projections in the monkey demonstrated by autoradiographic technics. The Journal of Comparative Neurology. 1976;**165**:401-415

[32] McGeorge AJ, Faull RL. The organization of the projection from the cerebral cortex to the striatum in the rat. Neuroscience. 1989;**29**:503-537

[33] Sadikot AF, Parent A, Smith Y, Bolam JP. Efferent connections of the centromedian and parafascicular thalamic nuclei in the squirrel monkey: A light and electron microscopic study of the thalamostriatal projection in relation to striatal heterogeneity. The Journal of Comparative Neurology. 1992;**320**:228-242

[34] Kawaguchi Y, Wilson CJ, Augood SJ, Emson PC. Striatal interneurones: Chemical, physiological and morphological characterization. Trends in Neurosciences. 1995;**18**:527-535

[35] Trottier Y, Lutz Y, Stevanin G, Imbert G, Devys D, Cancel G, et al. Polyglutamine expansion as a pathological epitope in Huntington's disease and four dominant cerebellar ataxias. Nature. 1995;**378**:403-406

[36] Vonsattel JPG, Difiglia M. Huntington disease. Journal of Neuropathology and Experimental Neurology. 1998;**57**:369-384

[37] Dawbarn D, De Quidt ME, Emson PC. Survival of basal ganglia neuropeptide Y-somatostatin neurones in Huntington's disease. Brain Research. 1985;**340**:251-260

[38] Ferrante RJ, Kowall NW, Beal MF, Richardson EP, Bird ED, Martin JB. Selective sparing of a class of striatal neurons in Huntington's disease. Science. 1985;**230**:561-563

[39] Reiner A, Shelby E, Wang H, Demarch Z, Deng Y, Guley NH, et al. Striatal parvalbuminergic neurons are lost in Huntington's disease: Implications for dystonia. Movement Disorders, The Official Journal of MDS. 2013;**28**:1691-1699

[40] Vonsattel JPG, Keller C, del Pilar Amaya M. Neuropathology of Huntington's disease. In: Handbook of Clinical Neurology. Amsterdam, Netherlands: Elsevier; 2008. pp. 599-618. Available from: https://www.sciencedirect.com/science/article/pii/S0072975207012560

[41] Vonsattel JP, Myers RH, Bird ED, Ge P, Richardson EJ. Huntington disease: 7 cases with relatively preserved neostriatal islets. Revue Neurologique (Paris). 1992;**148**:107-116

[42] Hickey MA, Chesselet MF. Apoptosis in Huntington's disease. Progress in Neuro-Psychopharmacology & Biological Psychiatry. 2003;**27**:255-265

[43] Rüb U, Vonsattel JPV, Heinsen H, Korf H-W. The neuropathology of Huntington's disease: Classical findings, recent developments and correlation to functional neuroanatomy. Advances in Anatomy, Embryology, and Cell Biology. 2015;**217**:1-146

[44] Ferrante RJ, Gutekunst C-A, Persichetti F, McNeil SM, Kowall NW, Gusella JF, et al. Heterogeneous topographic and cellular distribution of huntingtin expression in the Normal human Neostriatum. Journal of Neuroscience is an Official Journal of the Society for Neuroscience. 1997;**17**:3052-3063

[45] Ferrante RJ, Kowall NW, Beal MF, Martin JB, Bird ED, Richardson EP. Morphologic and histochemical characteristics of a spared subset of striatal neurons in Huntington's disease. Journal of Neuropathology and Experimental Neurology. 1987;**46**:12-27

[46] Seto-Ohshima A, Emson PC, Lawson E, Mountjoy CQ, Carrasco LH.

Loss of matrix calcium-binding protein-containing neurons in Huntington's disease. Lancet (London, England). 1988;**1**:1252-1255

[47] Hedreen JC, Folstein SE. Early loss of neostriatal striosome neurons in Huntington's disease. Journal of Neuropathology and Experimental Neurology. 1995;**54**:105-120

[48] Morton AJ, Nicholson LF, Faull RL. Compartmental loss of NADPH diaphorase in the neuropil of the human striatum in Huntington's disease. Neuroscience. 1993;**53**:159-168

[49] Tippett LJ, Waldvogel HJ, Thomas SJ, Hogg VM, van Roon-Mom W, Synek BJ, et al. Striosomes and mood dysfunction in Huntington's disease. Brain: A Journal of Neurology. 2007;**130**:206-221

[50] Augood SJ, Faull RL, Love DR, Emson PC. Reduction in enkephalin and substance P messenger RNA in the striatum of early grade Huntington's disease: A detailed cellular in situ hybridization study. Neuroscience. 1996;**72**:1023-1036

[51] Reiner A, Albin RL, Anderson KD, D'Amato CJ, Penney JB, Young AB. Differential loss of striatal projection neurons in Huntington disease. Proceedings of the National Academy of Sciences of the United States of America. 1988;**85**:5733-5737

[52] Deng YP, Albin RL, Penney JB, Young AB, Anderson KD, Reiner A. Differential loss of striatal projection systems in Huntington's disease: A quantitative immunohistochemical study. Journal of Chemical Neuroanatomy. 2004;**27**:143-164

[53] Gerfen CR, Engber TM, Mahan LC, Susel Z, Chase TN, Monsma FJ, et al. D1 and D2 dopamine receptor-regulated gene expression of striatonigral and striatopallidal neurons. Science. 1990;**250**:1429-1432

[54] Lange H, Thörner G, Hopf A, Schröder KF. Morphometric studies of the neuropathological changes in choreatic diseases. Journal of the Neurological Sciences. 1976;**28**:401-425

[55] Douaud G, Gaura V, Ribeiro M-J, Lethimonnier F, Maroy R, Verny C, et al. Distribution of grey matter atrophy in Huntington's disease patients: A combined ROI-based and voxel-based morphometric study. NeuroImage. 2006;**32**:1562-1575

[56] Guo Z, Rudow G, Pletnikova O, Codispoti K-E, Orr BA, Crain BJ, et al. Striatal neuronal loss correlates with clinical motor impairment in Huntington's disease. Movement Disorders, the Official Journal of MDS. 2012;**27**:1379-1386

[57] Campbell AM, Corner B, Norman RM, Urich H. The rigid form of Huntington's disease. Journal of Neurology, Neurosurgery, and Psychiatry. 1961;**24**:71-77

[58] Richardson EP. Huntington's disease: Some recent neuropathological studies. Neuropathology and Applied Neurobiology. 1990;**16**:451-460

[59] Oyanagi K, Ikuta F. A morphometric reevaluation of Huntington's chorea with special reference to the large neurons in the neostriatum. Clinical Neuropathology. 1987;**6**:71-79

[60] Oyanagi K, Takeda S, Takahashi H, Ohama E, Ikuta F. A quantitative investigation of the substantia nigra in Huntington's disease. Annals of Neurology. 1989;**26**:13-19

[61] Whitehouse PJ, Trifiletti RR, Jones BE, Folstein S, Price DL, Snyder SH, et al.

Neurotransmitter receptor alterations in Huntington's disease: Autoradiographic and homogenate studies with special reference to benzodiazepine receptor complexes. Annals of Neurology. 1985;**18**:202-210

[62] Young AB, Greenamyre JT, Hollingsworth Z, Albin R, D'Amato C, Shoulson I, et al. NMDA receptor losses in putamen from patients with Huntington's disease. Science. 1988;**241**:981-983

[63] Glass M, Dragunow M, Faull RL. The pattern of neurodegeneration in Huntington's disease: A comparative study of cannabinoid, dopamine, adenosine and GABA(a) receptor alterations in the human basal ganglia in Huntington's disease. Neuroscience. 2000;**97**:505-519

[64] Waters CM, Peck R, Rossor M, Reynolds GP, Hunt SP. Immunocyto chemical studies on the basal ganglia and substantia nigra in Parkinson's disease and Huntington's chorea. Neuroscience. 1988;**25**:419-438

[65] Handley RR, Reid SJ, Brauning R, Maclean P, Mears ER, Fourie I, et al. Brain urea increase is an early Huntington's disease pathogenic event observed in a prodromal transgenic sheep model and HD cases. Proceedings of the National Academy of Sciences of the United States of America. 2017;**114**:E11293-E11302

[66] Venco P, Dusi S, Valletta L, Tiranti V. Alteration of the coenzyme a biosynthetic pathway in neurodegeneration with brain iron accumulation syndromes. Biochemical Society Transactions. 2014;**42**:1069-1074

[67] Patassini S, Begley P, Xu J, Church SJ, Kureishy N, Reid SJ, et al. Cerebral vitamin B5 (D-pantothenic acid) deficiency as a potential cause of metabolic perturbation and neurodegeneration in Huntington's disease. Metabolites. 2019;**9**:113

[68] Cepeda C, Wu N, André VM, Cummings DM, Levine MS. The corticostriatal pathway in Huntington's disease. Progress in Neurobiology. 2007;**81**:253-271

[69] Cummings DM, André VM, Uzgil BO, Gee SM, Fisher YE, Cepeda C, et al. Alterations in cortical excitation and inhibition in genetic mouse models of Huntington's disease. Journal of Neuroscience: The Official Journal of the Society for Neuroscience. 2009;**29**:10371-10386

[70] Beal MF. Energetics in the pathogenesis of neurodegenerative diseases. Trends in Neurosciences. 2000;**23**:298-304

[71] Jiang R, Diaz-Castro B, Looger LL, Khakh BS. Dysfunctional calcium and glutamate Signaling in striatal astrocytes from Huntington's disease model mice. The Journal of Neuroscience. 2016;**36**:3453-3470

[72] Beal MF, Hyman BT, Koroshetz W. Do defecs in mitochondrial energy metabolism underlie the pathology of neurodegenerative diseases? Trends in Neurosciences. 1993;**16**:125-131

[73] Estrada Sánchez AM, Mejía-Toiber J, Massieu L. Excitotoxic neuronal death and the pathogenesis of Huntington's disease. Archives of Medical Research. 2008;**39**:265-276

[74] Kolodziejczyk K, Raymond LA. Differential changes in thalamic and cortical excitatory synapses onto striatal spiny projection neurons in a Huntington disease mouse model. Neurobiology of Disease. 2016;**86**:62-74

[75] Huang T-T, Smith R, Bacos K, Song D-Y, Faull RM, Waldvogel HJ, et al. No symphony without bassoon and piccolo: Changes in synaptic active zone proteins in Huntington's disease. Acta Neuropathologica Communications. 2020;**8**:77

[76] Terplan K. Zur pathologischen Anatomie der chronischen progressiven Chorea. Virchows Archiv fur pathologische Anatomie und Physiologie und fur klinische Medizin. 1924;**252**:146-176. Available from: https://link.springer.com/article/10.1007/BF01960725

[77] Dunlap CB. Pathologic changes in Huntington's chores: With special reference to the corpus striatum. Archives of Neurology and Psychiatry. 1927;**18**:867-943

[78] Rajkowska G, Selemon LD, Goldman-Rakic PS. Neuronal and glial somal size in the prefrontal cortex: A postmortem morphometric study of schizophrenia and Huntington disease. Archives of General Psychiatry. 1998;**55**:215-224

[79] Braak H, Braak E. The human entorhinal cortex: Normal morphology and lamina-specific pathology in various diseases. Neuroscience Research. 1992;**15**:6-31

[80] Hedreen JC, Peyser CE, Folstein SE, Ross CA. Neuronal loss in layers V and VI of cerebral cortex in Huntington's disease. Neuroscience Letters. 1991;**133**:257-261

[81] Cudkowicz M, Kowall NW. Degeneration of pyramidal projection neurons in Huntington's disease cortex. Annals of Neurology. 1990;**27**:200-204

[82] Macdonald V, Halliday G. Pyramidal cell loss in motor cortices in Huntington's disease. Neurobiology of Disease. 2002;**10**:378-386

[83] Thu DCV, Oorschot DE, Tippett LJ, Nana AL, Hogg VM, Synek BJ, et al. Cell loss in the motor and cingulate cortex correlates with symptomatology in Huntington's disease. Brain: A Journal of Neurology. 2010;**133**:1094-1110

[84] Sotrel A, Paskevich PA, Kiely DK, Bird ED, Williams RS, Myers RH. Morphometric analysis of the prefrontal cortex in Huntington's disease. Neurology. 1991;**41**:1117-1117

[85] Heinsen H, Strik M, Bauer M, Luther K, Ulmar G, Gangnus D, et al. Cortical and striatal neurone number in Huntington's disease. Acta Neuropathologica. 1994;**88**:320-333

[86] Montoya A, Price BH, Menear M, Lepage M. Brain imaging and cognitive dysfunctions in Huntington's disease. Journal of Psychiatry & Neuroscience. 2006;**31**:21-29

[87] Hobbs NZ, Pedrick AV, Say MJ, Frost C, Dar Santos R, Coleman A, et al. The structural involvement of the cingulate cortex in premanifest and early Huntington's disease. Movement Disorders, The Official Journal of MDS. 2011;**26**:1684-1690

[88] Manto M, Bower JM, Conforto AB, Delgado-García JM, da Guarda SNF, Gerwig M, et al. Consensus paper: Roles of the cerebellum in motor control—The diversity of ideas on cerebellar involvement in movement. The Cerebellum. 2012;**11**:457-487

[89] Middleton FA, Strick PL. The cerebellum: An overview. Trends in Neurosciences. 1998;**21**:367-369

[90] Paulin MG. The role of the cerebellum in motor control and perception.

Brain, Behavior and Evolution. 1993;**41**:39-50

[91] Rüb U, Hoche F, Brunt ER, Heinsen H, Seidel K, Del Turco D, et al. Degeneration of the cerebellum in Huntington's disease (HD): Possible relevance for the clinical picture and potential gateway to pathological mechanisms of the disease process. Brain Pathology. 2012;**23**:165-177

[92] Fennema-Notestine C, Archibald SL, Jacobson MW, Corey-Bloom J, Paulsen JS, Peavy GM, et al. In vivo evidence of cerebellar atrophy and cerebral white matter loss in Huntington disease. Neurology. 2004;**63**:989-995

[93] Singh-Bains MK, Mehrabi NF, Sehji T, Austria MDR, Tan AYS, Tippett LJ, et al. Cerebellar degeneration correlates with motor symptoms in Huntington disease. Annals of Neurology. 2019;**85**:396-405

[94] Lastres-Becker I, Rüb U, Auburger G. Spinocerebellar ataxia 2 (SCA2). Cerebellum (London, England). 2008;**7**:115-124

[95] Rüb U, Brunt ER, Deller T. New insights into the pathoanatomy of spinocerebellar ataxia type 3 (Machado-Joseph disease). Current Opinion in Neurology. 2008;**21**:111-116

[96] Rüb U, Brunt ER, Gierga K, Seidel K, Schultz C, Schöls L, et al. Spinocerebellar ataxia type 7 (SCA7): First report of a systematic neuropathological study of the brain of a patient with a very short expanded CAG-repeat. Brain Pathology (Zurich, Switzerland). 2005;**15**:287-295

[97] Margolis RL, Ross CA. Diagnosis of Huntington disease. Clinical Chemistry. 2003;**49**:1726-1732

[98] Koller WC, Trimble J. The gait abnormality of Huntington's disease. Neurology. 1985;**35**:1450-1454

[99] Lasker AG, Zee DS. Ocular motor abnormalities in Huntington's disease. Vision Research. 1997;**37**:3639-3645

[100] Kassubek J, Juengling FD, Ecker D, Landwehrmeyer GB. Thalamic atrophy in Huntington's disease co-varies with cognitive performance: A morphometric MRI analysis. Cerebral Cortex (New York, N.Y.) 1991. 2005;**15**:846-853

[101] Heinsen H, Rüb U, Gangnus D, Jungkunz G, Bauer M, Ulmar G, et al. Nerve cell loss in the thalamic centromedian-parafascicular complex in patients with Huntington's disease. Acta Neuropathologica. 1996;**91**:161-168

[102] Heinsen H, Rüb U, Bauer M, Ulmar G, Bethke B, Schüler M, et al. Nerve cell loss in the thalamic mediodorsal nucleus in Huntington's disease. Acta Neuropathologica. 1999;**97**:613-622

[103] Kassubek J, Gaus W, Landwehrmeyer GB. Evidence for more widespread cerebral pathology in early HD: An MRI-based morphometric analysis. Neurology. 2004;**62**:523-524; author reply 524

[104] Politis M, Pavese N, Tai YF, Tabrizi SJ, Barker RA, Piccini P. Hypothalamic involvement in Huntington's disease: An in vivo PET study. Brain: A Journal of Neurology. 2008;**131**:2860-2869

[105] van der Burg JMM, Björkqvist M, Brundin P. Beyond the brain: Widespread pathology in Huntington's disease. Lancet Neurology. 2009;**8**:765-774

[106] Morton AJ, Wood NI, Hastings MH, Hurelbrink C, Barker RA, Maywood ES. Disintegration of the sleep-wake cycle and circadian timing in Huntington's disease. Journal of Neuroscience: The Official Journal of the Society for Neuroscience. 2005;**25**:157-163

[107] Hult S, Schultz K, Soylu R, Petersén A. Hypothalamic and neuroendocrine changes in Huntington's disease. Current Drug Targets. 2010;**11**:1237-1249

[108] Aziz A, Fronczek R, Maat-Schieman M, Unmehopa U, Roelandse F, Overeem S, et al. Hypocretin and melanin-concentrating hormone in patients with Huntington disease. Brain Pathology (Zurich, Switzerland). 2008;**18**:474-483

[109] Timmers HJ, Swaab DF, van de Nes JA, Kremer HP. Somatostatin 1-12 immunoreactivity is decreased in the hypothalamic lateral tuberal nucleus of Huntington's disease patients. Brain Research. 1996;**728**:141-148

[110] Petersén A, Gil J, Maat-Schieman MLC, Björkqvist M, Tanila H, Araújo IM, et al. Orexin loss in Huntington's disease. Human Molecular Genetics. 2005;**14**:39-47

[111] Stephen CD, Hung J, Schifitto G, Hersch SM, Rosas HD. Electrocardiogram abnormalities suggest aberrant cardiac conduction in Huntington's disease. Movement Disorders Clinical Practice. 2018;**5**:306-311

[112] Spargo E, Everall IP, Lantos PL. Neuronal loss in the hippocampus in Huntington's disease: A comparison with HIV infection. Journal of Neurology, Neurosurgery, and Psychiatry. 1993;**56**:487-491

[113] Curtis MA, Penney EB, Pearson AG, van Roon-Mom WMC, Butterworth NJ, Dragunow M, et al. Increased cell proliferation and neurogenesis in the adult human Huntington's disease brain. Proceedings of the National Academy of Sciences of the United States of America. 2003;**100**:9023-9027

[114] Hunter M, Demarais NJ, Faull RLM, Grey AC, Curtis MA. Subventricular zone lipidomic architecture loss in Huntington's disease. Journal of Neurochemistry. 2018;**146**:613-630

[115] Rosas HD, Lee SY, Bender AC, Zaleta AK, Vangel M, Yu P, et al. Altered white matter microstructure in the corpus callosum in Huntington's disease: Implications for cortical "disconnection.". NeuroImage. 2010;**49**:2995-3004

[116] Rosas HD, Tuch DS, Hevelone ND, Zaleta AK, Vangel M, Hersch SM, et al. Diffusion tensor imaging in presymptomatic and early Huntington's disease: Selective white matter pathology and its relationship to clinical measures. Movement Disorders, the official Journal of MDS. 2006;**21**:1317-1325

[117] Rüb U, Heinsen H, Brunt ER, Landwehrmeyer B, Den Dunnen WFA, Gierga K, et al. The human premotor oculomotor brainstem system—Can it help to understand oculomotor symptoms in Huntington's disease? Neuropathology and Applied Neurobiology. 2009;**35**:4-15

[118] Grinberg L, Rueb U, Heinsen H. Brainstem: Neglected locus in neurodegenerative diseases. Frontiers in Neurology. 2011;**2**:1-9. Available from: https://www.frontiersin.org/article/10.3389/fneur.2011.00042

[119] Andrich J, Schmitz T, Saft C, Postert T, Kraus P, Epplen J, et al.

Autonomic nervous system function in Huntington's disease. Journal of Neurology, Neurosurgery, and Psychiatry. 2002;**72**:726-731

[120] Hoffner G, Souès S, Djian P. Aggregation of expanded huntingtin in the brains of patients with Huntington disease. Prion. 2007;**1**:26-31

[121] Perutz MF. Glutamine repeats and inherited neurodegenerative diseases: Molecular aspects. Current Opinion in Structural Biology. 1996;**6**:848-858

[122] Perutz MF, Johnson T, Suzuki M, Finch JT. Glutamine repeats as polar zippers: Their possible role in inherited neurodegenerative diseases. Proceedings of the National Academy of Sciences of the United States of America. 1994;**91**:5355-5358

[123] Gutekunst C-A, Li S-H, Yi H, Mulroy JS, Kuemmerle S, Jones R, et al. Nuclear and neuropil aggregates in Huntington's disease: Relationship to neuropathology. The Journal of Neuroscience. 1999;**19**:2522-2534

[124] Waldvogel HJ, Kim EH, Tippett LJ, Vonsattel J-PG, Faull RL. The neuropathology of Huntington's disease. In: Nguyen HHP, Cenci MA, editors. Behav Neurobiol Huntingt Dis Park Dis. Berlin, Heidelberg: Springer; 2015. p. 33-80. 10.1007/7854_2014_354

[125] Jansen AHP, van Hal M, op den Kelder IC, Meier RT, de Ruiter A-A, Schut MH, et al. Frequency of nuclear mutant huntingtin inclusion formation in neurons and glia is cell-type-specific. Glia. 2017;**65**:50-61

[126] Shin J-Y, Fang Z-H, Yu Z-X, Wang C-E, Li S-H, Li X-J. Expression of mutant huntingtin in glial cells contributes to neuronal excitotoxicity. The Journal of Cell Biology. 2005;**171**:1001-1012

[127] Gómez-Tortosa E, MacDonald ME, Friend JC, Taylor SA, Weiler LJ, Cupples LA, et al. Quantitative neuropathological changes in presymptomatic Huntington's disease [internet]. Annals of Neurology. 2001;**49**:29-34. Available from: https://onlinelibrary.wiley.com/doi/full/10.1002/1531-8249%28200101%2949%3A1%3C29%3A%3AAID-ANA7%3E3.0.CO%3B2-B?casa_token=8vbK8PmpnjEAAAAA%3ArqcpW7Iudk21Tf-7SgXDb9pZM35BlDFh2RB0ajIwHlBrpjrdTgpJ0C9UZ9t5GrC2f4_k0joBOFsr0Rs

[128] Highet B, Dieriks BV, Murray HC, Faull RLM, Curtis MA. Huntingtin aggregates in the olfactory bulb in Huntington's disease. Frontiers in Aging Neuroscience. 2020;**12**:261

[129] Herndon ES, Hladik CL, Shang P, Burns DK, Raisanen J, White CL III. Neuroanatomic profile of polyglutamine immunoreactivity in Huntington disease brains. Journal of Neuropathology and Experimental Neurology. 2009;**68**:250-261

[130] Gourfinkel-An I, Cancel G, Duyckaerts C, Faucheux B, Hauw J-J, Trottier Y, et al. Neuronal distribution of intranuclear inclusions in Huntington's disease with adult onset. Neuroreport. 1998;**9**:1823-1826

[131] Djoussé L, Knowlton B, Cupples LA, Marder K, Shoulson I, Myers RH. Weight loss in early stage of Huntington's disease. Neurology. 2002;**59**:1325-1330

[132] Lanska DJ, Lanska MJ, Lavine L, Schoenberg BS. Conditions associated with Huntington's disease at death: A case-control study. Archives of Neurology. 1988;**45**:878-880

[133] Van Raamsdonk JM, Murphy Z, Selva DM, Hamidizadeh R, Pearson J,

Åsa P, et al. Testicular degeneration in Huntington disease. Neurobiology of Disease. 2007;**26**:512-520

[134] Trejo A, Tarrats RM, MaE A, Boll M-C, Ochoa A, Velásquez L. Assessment of the nutrition status of patients with Huntington's disease. Nutrition. 2004;**20**:192-196

[135] Orth M, Cooper JM, Bates GP, Schapira AHV. Inclusion formation in Huntington's disease R6/2 mouse muscle cultures. Journal of Neurochemistry. 2003;**87**:1-6

[136] Kojer K, Hering T, Bazenet C, Weiss A, Herrmann F, Taanman J-W, et al. Huntingtin aggregates and mitochondrial pathology in skeletal muscle but not heart of late-stage R6/2 mice. Journal of Huntington's Disease. 2019;**8**:145-159

[137] Ciammola A, Sassone J, Alberti L, Meola G, Mancinelli E, Russo MA, et al. Increased apoptosis, huntingtin inclusions and altered differentiation in muscle cell cultures from Huntington's disease subjects. Cell Death and Differentiation. 2006;**13**:2068-2078

[138] Arenas J, Campos Y, Ribacoba R, Martín MA, Rubio JC, Ablanedo P, et al. Complex I defect in muscle from patients with Huntington's disease. Annals of Neurology. 1998;**43**:397-400

[139] Turner C, Cooper JM, Schapira AHV. Clinical correlates of mitochondrial function in Huntington's disease muscle. Movement Disorders. 2007;**22**:1715-1721

[140] Sathasivam K, Hobbs C, Turmaine M, Mangiarini L, Mahal A, Bertaux F, et al. Formation of polyglutamine inclusions in non-CNS tissue. Human Molecular Genetics. 1999;**8**:813-822

[141] Bär KJ, Boettger MK, Andrich J, Epplen JT, Fischer F, Cordes J, et al. Cardiovagal modulation upon postural change is altered in Huntington's disease. European Journal of Neurology. 2008;**15**:869-871

[142] Dridi H, Liu X, Yuan Q, Reiken S, Yehya M, Sittenfeld L, et al. Role of defective calcium regulation in cardiorespiratory dysfunction in Huntington's disease. JCI Insight. 2020;**5**:1-21. Available from: https://insight.jci.org/articles/view/140614

[143] Palpagama TH, Waldvogel HJ, Faull RLM, Kwakowsky A. The role of microglia and astrocytes in Huntington's disease. Frontiers in Molecular Neuroscience. 2019;**12**:1-15. Available from: https://www.frontiersin.org/article/10.3389/fnmol.2019.00258

[144] Myers RH, Vonsattel JP, Paskevich PA, Kiely DK, Stevens TJ, Cupples LA, et al. Decreased neuronal and increased oligodendroglial densities in Huntington's disease caudate nucleus. Journal of Neuropathology and Experimental Neurology. 1991;**50**:729-742

[145] Sapp E, Kegel KB, Aronin N, Hashikawa T, Uchiyama Y, Tohyama K, et al. Early and progressive accumulation of reactive microglia in the Huntington disease brain. Journal of Neuropathology and Experimental Neurology. 2001;**60**:161-172

[146] Pavese N, Gerhard A, Tai YF, Ho AK, Turkheimer F, Barker RA, et al. Microglial activation correlates with severity in Huntington disease: A clinical and PET study. Neurology. 2006;**66**:1638-1643

[147] Tai YF, Pavese N, Gerhard A, Tabrizi SJ, Barker RA, Brooks DJ, et al. Imaging microglial activation in

Huntington's disease. Brain Research Bulletin. 2007;**72**:148-151

[148] Tai YF, Pavese N, Gerhard A, Tabrizi SJ, Barker RA, Brooks DJ, et al. Microglial activation in presymptomatic Huntington's disease gene carriers. Brain. 2007;**130**:1759-1766

[149] Miller SJ. Astrocyte heterogeneity in the adult central nervous system. Frontiers in Cellular Neuroscience. 2018;**12**:1-6. Available from: https://www.frontiersin.org/article/10.3389/fncel.2018.00401

[150] Hasel P, Rose IVL, Sadick JS, Kim RD, Liddelow SA. Neuroinflammatory astrocyte subtypes in the mouse brain. Nature Neuroscience. 2021;**24**:1-13

[151] Al-Dalahmah O, Sosunov AA, Shaik A, Ofori K, Liu Y, Vonsattel JP, et al. Single-nucleus RNA-seq identifies Huntington disease astrocyte states. Acta Neuropathologica Communications. 2020;**8**:19

[152] Liddelow SA, Barres BA. Reactive astrocytes: Production, function, and therapeutic potential. Immunity. 2017;**46**:957-967

[153] Markham CH, Knox JW. Oberservations on Huntington's chorea in childhood. The Journal of Pediatrics. 1965;**67**:46-57

[154] Oliver J, Dewhurst K. Childhood and adolescent forms of Huntington's disease. Journal of Neurology, Neurosurgery, and Psychiatry. 1969;**32**:455-459

[155] Latimer CS, Flanagan ME, Cimino PJ, Jayadev S, Davis M, Hoffer ZS, et al. Neuropathological comparison of adult onset and juvenile Huntington's disease with cerebellar atrophy: A report of a father and son. Journal of Huntington's Disease. 2017;**6**:337-348

[156] Fusilli C, Migliore S, Mazza T, Consoli F, Luca AD, Barbagallo G, et al. Biological and clinical manifestations of juvenile Huntington's disease: A retrospective analysis. Lancet Neurology. 2018;**17**:986-993

[157] Bakels HS, Roos RAC, van Roon-Mom WMC, de Bot ST. Juvenile-onset Huntington disease pathophysiology and neurodevelopment: A review. Movement Disorders. 2022;**37**:16-24

[158] Byers RK, Gilles FH, Fung C. Huntington's disease in children: Neuropathologic study of four cases. Neurology. 1973;**23**:561-561

[159] Vonsattel JPG, Cortes EP, Keller CE. Juvenile Huntington's disease: Neuropathology [Internet]. Juvenile Huntington Disease. 2022;**5**:52-78. Available from: https://oxfordmedicine-com.ezp1.lib.umn.edu/view/10.1093/med/9780199236121.001.0001/med-9780199236121-chapter-5

[160] Ruocco HH, Bonilha L, Li LM, Lopes-Cendes I, Cendes F. Longitudinal analysis of regional grey matter loss in Huntington disease: Effects of the length of the expanded CAG repeat. Journal of Neurology, Neurosurgery, and Psychiatry. 2008;**79**:130-135

[161] Barnat M, Capizzi M, Aparicio E, Boluda S, Wennagel D, Kacher R, et al. Huntington's disease alters human neurodevelopment. Science. 2020;**369**:787-793

[162] Mangin J-F, Rivière D, Duchesnay E, Cointepas Y, Gaura V, Verny C, et al. Neocortical morphometry

in Huntington's disease: Indication of the coexistence of abnormal neurodevelopmental and neurodegenerative processes. NeuroImage: Clinical. 2020;**26**:102211

[163] Tereshchenko AV, Schultz JL, Bruss JE, Magnotta VA, Epping EA, Nopoulos PC. Abnormal development of cerebellar-striatal circuitry in Huntington disease. Neurology. 2020;**94**:e1908-e1915

[164] van der Plas E, Langbehn DR, Conrad AL, Koscik TR, Tereshchenko A, Epping EA, et al. Abnormal brain development in child and adolescent carriers of mutant huntingtin. Neurology. 2019;**93**:e1021-e1030

[165] Hickman RA, Faust PL, Rosenblum MK, Marder K, Mehler MF, Vonsattel JP. Developmental malformations in Huntington disease: Neuropathologic evidence of focal neuronal migration defects in a subset of adult brains. Acta Neuropathologica. 2021;**141**:399-413

Chapter 3

Exploring Biomarkers for Huntington's Disease

Omar Deeb, Afnan Atallah and Sawsan Salameh

Abstract

Huntington's disease (HD) is a progressive, non-curative, autosomal dominant neurodegenerative disease characterized by prominent psychiatric problems, as well as progressive deterioration in both cognitive function and motor control. The success of therapeutic interventions in HD patients cannot be easily examined without reliable and practical measurements by using effective biomarkers. Many clinical trials have been held to evaluate biomarkers efficacies in disease-modifying treatment before the manifestation of the disease or its severity. Biofluid (wet) biomarkers have potential advantages of direct quantification of biological processes at the molecular level, imaging biomarkers, on the other hand, can quantify related changes at a structural level in the brain. The most robust biofluid and imaging biomarkers are being investigated for their clinical use and development of future treatment and can offer complementary information, providing a more comprehensive evaluation of disease stage and progression.

Keywords: Huntington's disease (HD), biomarkers, clinical biomarkers, wet biomarkers, imaging biomarkers, premanifest, manifest

1. Introduction

Huntington's disease (HD) is an inherited disease that causes breakdown of nerve cells in the brain. HD, resulting from gene mutation, affects different parts of the brain impacting movement, behavior, emotion regulation, and psychiatric disturbance. Eventually, the person will need full-time care, and death of the disease is inescapable. HD is caused by an expanded trinucleotide cytosine-adenine-guanine (CAG) repeat in the huntingtin gene. HD is one of the rare neurodegenerative conditions for which predictive genetic testing is available for individuals with a known family history [1]. The identification of HD gene mutation carriers, while they are still healthy before manifestation (premanifest) of clinical signs of the disease has several benefits as this may help prevent the development or slowdown of the progression of the disease, hence, improved quality of life of the patient.

HD symptoms can develop at any time, but they often start at 30–50 years of age. If the condition develops earlier, before the age of 20, the symptoms start with behavioral disturbances and learning difficulties. Because of this, there is an urgent need to diagnose the disease as early as possible using biomarkers and assess the development of the disease. This can be achieved by identifying a number of biomarkers that are altered either premanifest or during the disease progression.

IntechOpen

The unified Huntington's Rating Scale (UHDRS) has been used as a clinical rating scale to assess four domains (motor function, cognitive function, behavioral abnormalities, and functional capacity) of clinical performance and capacity in HD patients. However, one of the main challenges in using this rating scale is the slow progression of HD, rendering the scale imperfect as a standalone tool [2] leading, in some cases, to limitations of clinical trials that aiming to assess the benefits of therapeutic agents in HD. In addition, there are several factors that could influence the clinical measures including the placebo effect and the clinical rater variability. This results in reduced ability indistinguishing between symptom relief and amelioration of the underlying disease process [3].

Finding biomarkers that change with clinical progression quickly and predictably with the use of a therapeutic agent could greatly facilitate future HD clinical trials by reducing the duration and number of patient volunteer required for such studies. This is especially important in premanifest HD mutation carriers, who may remain free from all clinical manifestations for decades. In addition, pharmacodynamic biomarkers can be utilized in preclinical trials and early phase clinical trials to predict if the therapeutic agent will have its intended effect and to assist in the decision-making process on whether to continue such trials or not.

Up to date biomarker research has included both focused small-scale and large studies. For instance, TRACK-HD (a prospective observational study of HD that examines disease progression in premanifest individuals carrying the mutant HTT gene and those with early-stage disease and those who have had it for 12 months or less) [4], and PREDICT-HD (a multicenter observational research study aimed to examine measures that may be associated with disease in the largest cohort ever recruited of pre-diagnosed individuals carrying the gene expansion for HD) [5], have afforded scientists in the field the opportunity to study many potential biomarkers for HD.

2. Biomarkers

The term biomarker is defined as "a characteristic that is objectively measured and evaluated as an indicator of normal biological processes, pathogenic processes, or pharmacologic responses to a therapeutic intervention" [6]. Therefore, a biomarker can be related to the disease itself or to the response to treatment. Hence, biomarkers can serve many different functions, such as diagnostic, prognostic, monitoring, response/pharmacodynamic, susceptibility/Risk Biomarker [7, 8]. In addition, most therapeutic clinical trials that aim to evaluate the efficacy of potential disease-modifying treatments during pre-manifest HD require biomarkers to serve as outcome measures. Some efficacy biomarkers may also function as 'state biomarkers' or 'biomarkers of progression', which are used as indicators of disease severity. These state biomarkers could very well reflect the underlying disease pathobiology and linearly track clinical progression of the disease (including during the pre-manifest stage) [1].

The biomarkers that have been used, hitherto, in HD are of types including, clinical biomarkers, wet biomarkers, and imaging biomarkers. Detailed discussion of these biomarkers and their subtypes is presented below.

2.1 Clinical biomarkers

Rather than relying on United Huntington's Disease Rating Scale (UHDRS's) dichotomous notion of 'disease onset', some researchers have proposed the use of continuous measures, such as clinical symptoms of the disease. Some UHDRS motor abnormalities can be objectively quantified, thereby improving accuracy and reducing inter-rater and intra-rater variability [1].

Tabrizi et al. have supported the hypothesis that neuronal dysfunction occurs many years before the development of motor signs that are diagnostic of HD. The motor alterations that have been described are most likely secondary to progressive neuronal loss or dysfunction. This could help define quantifiable endpoints for future therapeutic interventions [9]. Motor signs are amenable to quantitative assessment and may provide objective measures for disease onset and progression. Several quantitative motor tasks, including force-transducer-based assessments, detect deficits in premanifest gene carriers [10], for example, finger tapping precision and a problem task is evident even in pre-manifest HD and worsen with time. Another longitudinal study identified numerous cognitive task impairments in more than one variable, one of these variables is the Symbol Digit Modalities test which assesses visual attention and psychomotor speed [1, 10, 11] suggesting the limited use of clinical markers in preventive clinical trials.

2.2 Wet biomarkers

Wet biomarkers also called biofluids, (those obtained from bodily fluids, such as blood, urine, saliva, and cerebrospinal fluids (CSF)) are another potential source of useful outcome measures if they reflect the pathophysiology of a disease and show the response for a therapeutic agent.

In HD, various pathologic mechanisms have been implicated and numerous potential molecular markers have been detected. Progression of the disease have been reported to be associated with detectable changes in inflammatory signals in peripheral blood which matched changes in peripheral and central processes such as immune activation, neuroinflammation, and metabolic markers [12, 13]. In some cases, substances that are released from dying neurons that can penetrate the blood-brain barrier can be detected in peripheral blood and could be used as a biomarker. Unfortunately, however, if these substances have peripheral sources, conflict in interpretation may occur [14]. Cerebrospinal fluid, which is enriched with brain-derived substances is of particular interest, however, other biofluids have the potential to yield relevant biomarkers if their composition reflects that of the CNS. Consequently, all biofluids, including CSF, may reflect peripheral as well as central disease-related changes [3].

2.2.1 Mutant huntingtin protein

Huntington's disease (HD) is caused by a cytosine-adenine-guanine (CAG) trinucleotide repeat expansion in the huntingtin gene (HTT), which leads to the production of the mutant huntingtin (mHTT) protein. The degree of symptom severity, disease stage, and markers of neuronal damage have been shown to correlate with levels of mHTT protein in the CSF in patients with HD. This toxic mHTT protein production is believed to result in neurotoxicity, as normal cellular processes important for cellular survival are disrupted. Furthermore, decreased level of mHTT is an important measure of the response to the therapeutic agents. mHTT quantification has been achieved for the first time in 2015 using a `femtomolar` single molecule counting (SMC) immunoassay, and a combination of mHTT N-terminal-detecting 2B7 antibody and polyglutamine-binding MW1 antibody. mHTT was significantly higher in manifest HD and premanifest HD compared to controls with a roughly threefold difference seen between premanifest HD and manifest [3, 14].

mHTT detection is associated with disease onset and cognitive and motor function disability. mHTT quantification in CSF could potentially serve as a biomarker for the development and testing of experimental mHTT-lowering therapies for HD [15]. mHTT levels also correlate with clinical manifestations as well as with two indicators of neuronal damage (CSF tau and neurofilament light chain) [14] suggesting that mHTT is released from damaged or dying neurons.

2.2.2 Neurofilament light and tau protein

Neurofilament light protein (NfL, also known as NFL) is the smallest of three subunits that make up neurofilaments, which are major components of the neuronal cytoskeleton. NfL is released from damaged neurons. Its concentrations in CSF are elevated in people with neurodegenerative diseases.

Detection of NfL in the CSF using enzyme-linked immunosorbent assay (ELISA) reflects that NfL concentration is elevated in both premanifest and manifest HD. This elevation is associated with mHTT elevation in CSF, disease stage, motor and cognitive impairment, functional impairment and brain atrophy, as well as reduction in all brain volume measures [14, 16–18].

Also, NfL is detectable in blood plasma or serum using a single-molecule 'Simoa' assay. It has been shown to increase in blood of people with neurodegenerative diseases including HD [14, 16]. Quantification of NfL in plasma provides an accessible biomarker that has close links to diagnosis, progression of HD and the response to disease-modifying treatments. Also, NfL in both plasma and CSF is considered a better biomarker to differentiate between premanifest and manifest HD than CSF mHTT [3, 17–19].

Tau protein (a microtubule-associated protein, which aggregates abnormally under certain pathologic conditions) is another protein that is hypothesized to be associated withHD. It has been found that CSF tau concentration in HD gene mutation carriers is increased compared with that of healthy controls. It has also been reported that CSF tau concentrations are associated with phenotypic variability in HD. This report strengthens the case for CSF tau as a biomarker in HD [20].

2.2.3 Inflammatory markers

Activation of glial cells has been reported in several neurodegenerative diseases including HD. Biomarkers reflecting these peripheral and/or central neuroinflammation could be useful to identify the disease onset, progression, and the therapeutic response. Proteomics screen of HD plasma identified immune proteins that are elevated in HD compared to healthy controls, including pro-inflammatory cytokine IL-6, acute-phase protein alpha-2-macroglobulin, complement factors, and a complement inhibitor clusterin. Additionally, it has been found that IL-6 levels were significantly increased in premanifest subjects with an estimated mean of 16 years before motor signs onset [8, 12, 16, 21].

Another marker that has also been studied as a CSF inflammatory marker in HD is YKL-40 (chitinase 3-like protein 1 (CHI3L1)), a member of the glycosyl hydrolase family 18 and a marker of microglial activation. The results about this marker are mixed [3, 14, 16].

2.2.4 Metabolic markers

Weight loss and muscle wasting are examples of some disorders that appear in patients with HD reflecting metabolic alterations in those patients. Several metabolites were tested as potential biomarkers for HD. In addition, several amino acids were tested as potential biomarkers. It has been reported that plasma levels of asparagine (Asn) and Serine (Ser) were significantly decreased suggesting a potential biomarker role for these two amino acids [22].

Studies conducted on the association of total cholesterol, HDL-cholesterol and LDL-cholesterol with HD revealed mixed, and in some cases, contradictory results. Whereas most studies showed that changes in cholesterol levels were insignificant, one study showed that reductions in cholesterol levels were significant in premanifest and manifest patients [23]. In another study, 24(S) hydroxycholesterol (24OHC), the brain-specific elimination product of cholesterol long considered a marker of brain cholesterol turnover, was significantly reduced in HD patients at all disease stages. This reduction was paralleled with a reduction of the caudate volume suggesting that the reduction of 24OHC may reflect progressive neuronal loss in HD patients. In addition, a decrease in the plasma concentration of cholesterol precursors` lanosterol and lathosterol was observed [8, 24, 25]. These results suggest the potential usefulness of these two cholesterol precursors as metabolic biomarkers in HD diagnosis and progression.

2.2.5 Neuroendocrine markers

Patients with manifest HD display circadian rhythm abnormalities with disturbances in rest-activity profiles and abnormal day-night ratios associated with alterations in sleep-wake timing and melatonin and cortisol profiles [26].

Melatonin is a light-sensitive hormone secreted predominantly by the pineal gland and displays a circadian rhythm with maximum levels peaking at night. It has a key role in the sleep-wake cycle which is disrupted in the early stages of HD. A significant decrease in mean melatonin levels has been reported in manifest HD, with trends towards decreased melatonin levels in premanifest HD and temporal shift in melatonin release in mHTT carriers. Altered melatonin patterns may provide an explanation for disrupted sleep and circadian behavior of HD patients acting as a biomarker for this disease state [3, 26–29]. While there were no differences in melatonin release when it was measured at a single time point in advanced HD, differences in melatonin release were detected when measured at multiple time points. This suggests the need to measure melatonin levels at points representing the whole circadian rhythmicity [8].

Cortisol is another substance that plays a role in circadian rhythm as it has been observed that increased cortisol levels lead to sleep disturbances, which are likely to potentiate neurodegeneration and associated changes in cognitive, motor deficits and mood disturbances in HD [27, 30].

With markers that have specific circadian rhythms, 24-hour sample collections could be the means to using these markers as pharmacodynamic markers to assess the response to the treatment rather than the progression of the disease [3].

2.2.6 Oxidative stress markers

Both human and animal studies have suggested the involvement of energy metabolism dysfunction and oxidative stress in HD pathogenesis as it has been shown that levels of oxidative damage products, free radical production are elevated in areas of degeneration in HD brain [31]. It is thought that impairment in the electron transport chain and mitochondrial dysfunction are behind the increased production of reactive oxygen species in HD [32–34]. Markers of oxidative stress have been investigated in HD blood plasma and brain tissue in the animal model, but few have been quantified in CSF.

Several studies have reported enhanced lipid peroxidation in individuals with HD with a correlation between lipid peroxidation products in plasma and the degree of severity in patients with HD. It has been reported that F2-isoprostanes are a marker for lipid peroxidation found to be elevated in HD [3, 8, 14].

2.2.7 Endogenous opioid peptides

The endogenous opioid peptides have been found to be implicated in the regulation of motor function as well as in the pathophysiology of abnormal movement disorders. Degeneration of opioid peptide-containing neurons in the basal ganglia has been demonstrated in some neurodegenerative diseases such as HD [35]. Recently, it has been found that CSF proenkephalin (PENK) levels were significantly decreased in manifest HD patients compared to premanifest. The decrease in PENK CSF levels in premanifest patients was insignificant when compared to controls. Moreover, levels of PENK in the CSF is inversely proportional to the progression of HD symptoms. This decrease in PENK levels reflects the degeneration or dysfunction of neurons that produce PENK, consequently, PENK levels may serve as marker for the state of medium spiny neurons (MSNs) in HD patients [36].

Prodynorphin (PDYN) is another endogenous opioid that has been studied in HD. It has been found that PDYN-derived peptide levels were significantly decreased in CSF of patients with HD. This decrease is unique to HD as a comparable decrease was not observed in the other neurodegenerative disorders studied. These results suggest that PDYN-derived peptides in CSF could be considered as strong biomarker candidates for HD [37].

2.2.8 MicroRNAs

The microRNAs (miRNAs) are involved in different biological processes including development, proliferation, inflammation and apoptosis. miRNA is an intracellular component but also can be detected in the peripheral circulation. The level, structure, type and sequence of miRNAs detected in blood will reflect the physiological status, the type and stage of the disease [38]. The detection of abnormal expression of different miRNAs in the HD mouse model provides further support regarding the importance of miRNA in HD pathogenesis and therapeutics [39], and the potential usefulness of miRNAs as biomarkers for diagnosis, prognosis, and therapeutic response [38].

2.2.9 Exosomes

In the central nervous system (CNS), exosomes play essential physiological roles in the cell-to-cell communication and homeostasis maintenance required for normal brain function [40]. Exosomes contain a variety of key bioactive substances reflecting the status of the intracellular environment. As exosomes can penetrate the blood-brain barrier they can be found in peripheral body fluids, and their contents will change with diseases [41]. Most cell types in the brain release extracellular vesicles (EVs) and these have been shown to contain neurodegenerative proteins. In HD, by using a model culture system with overexpression of HTT-exon 1 polyQ-GFP constructs in human 293 T cells, it has been found that the EVs did incorporate both the polyQ-GFP protein as well as the expanded repeat RNA. These findings support the role of EVs as delivery vehicles of toxic expanded trinucleotide repeat RNAs from one cell to another [42]. Exosomes have a huge potential as non-invasive diagnostic biomarkers of HD for their content of mHTT, its fragments, or other proteins reflect the conditions of exosomes producing CNS cells [40].

2.3 Imaging biomarkers

In HD, neuroimaging techniques have been extensively investigated and have aided in our understanding of the disease's natural history. Imaging is attractive as a source of biomarkers because it is generally non-invasive; data collecting, processing, and quality control can be standardized, and data can be easily sent over great distances, which is advantageous for multi-site investigations. The ideal imaging biomarker would be widely available, reasonably priced, and repeatable across multiple sites using different scanner manufacturers and field strengths and have a reasonable acquisition time - especially since HD patients may not tolerate longer scanning protocols and movement that degrades image quality.

Structural MRI, diffusion imaging, functional MRI, and PET are just a few of the imaging modalities available. There are a variety of image processing algorithms for each modality, and the approach chosen can have a big impact on the output metrics that are used as biomarkers. Some automated procedures, for example, can generate mistake and systemic bias, especially in atrophic brains [43]. To avoid difficulties, extensive validation of the acquisition and processing technique is essential before such measures may be used as a biomarker, which has been absent in many imaging investigations to date.

2.3.1 Structural volumetric MRI

Structural MRI (sMRI) is a non-invasive technique that provides information to describe the shape, size, and integrity of gray and white matter structures in the brain. MRI results emphasized that there are strong correlations between many gray and white matter regions and clinical tests, including recognition of negative emotions, metronome tapping precision, and measures of tongue force. The latest findings point of sMRI data enables to collect information from across the brain during the premanifest to manifest period in HD. The data show that no uniform atrophy occurs throughout the brain (**Figure 1**), where the largest changes (~18–22%) occurring in the striatum (caudate, pallidum, and putamen) and gradual changes (~7–16%) occurring across the four main brain regions (parietal, temporal, frontal, and occipital) over a period of ~11 years [44]. This timeframe is similar to prior studies of the timing of sMRI alterations in HD [45], according to which the rate of putamen and caudate atrophy becomes substantial roughly 9 and 11 years after estimated onset, respectively [44].

When used as a clinical trial endpoint, the rate of change of a proposed biomarker can influence the length of the study and the number of participants required to identify a meaningful change. There is no agreement on whether the pace of striatal atrophy progression differs with disease stage. TRACK-HD found stepwise

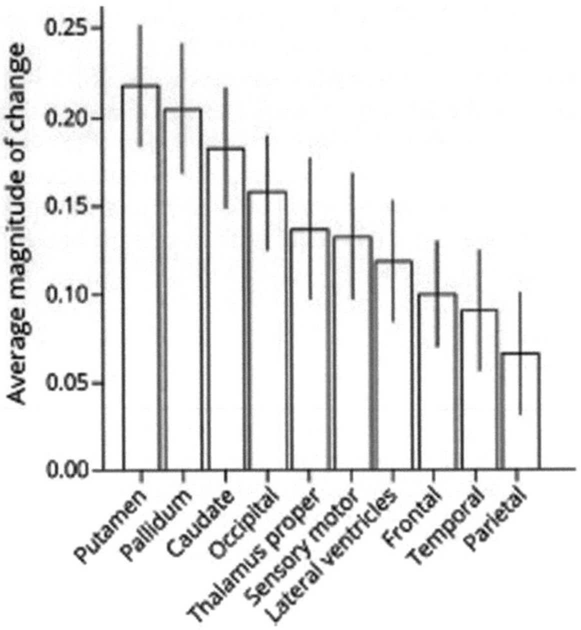

Figure 1.
RACK-HD cohort. Average magnitude of change of ten regional volumes from genotype-positive trajectories in TRACK-HD [44].

accelerated rates of change from the earliest premanifest stage to early-stage disease, with limited evidence that the acceleration diminishes after symptoms appear [4, 46]. After controlling for age, TRACK-HD found highly significant relationships between the rate of change and disease burden ratings in both the caudate and putamen. The PREDICT-HD study, on the other hand, did not discover that rates accelerated across its premanifest group, but this could be due to differences in longitudinal change assessment methodology [47].

Studies for regional Cortical found in HD patients reported a heterogeneous volume loss [4, 9, 46, 48–50], where the cortical thinning occurs early during the clinical stage of disease and seems to increase with disease progression. The reported thinning of the cortical gray was clear in posterior cortical regions, with increasing duration of symptoms, more anterior cortical regions were affected. The reported data suggest that the cortex undergoes degeneration, much of which occurs in the striatum particularly in the early premanifest stage of the disease [46, 48, 51]. Cortical thinning was distributed in many areas, even within gray regions. In some areas the thinning was as much as 0.4 mm which corresponds to approximately a 20% loss of thickness whereas in other areas, thinning was around 1 mm, corresponding to 30% loss of thickness (**Figure 2**) [49, 53–57].

The Cross-sectional studies have reported volume reductions in the corpus callosum [5] and frontal white matter (**Figure 3**) [9, 52, 59]. In premanifest HD, both TRACK-HD and PREDICT-HD showed progressive white matter atrophy, even in the groups farthest from anticipated onset [9, 46, 60]. In manifest disease, a similar picture has been observed, with cross-sectional reductions in white matter volume compared to controls [4, 9, 61–63], and elevated atrophy rates in longitudinal studies [52, 64]. White matter atrophy has been shown to correlate with motor function [47, 59, 65, 66], cognitive function [59, 65, 67] and total functional capacity (TFC) [47, 68]. White matter volume

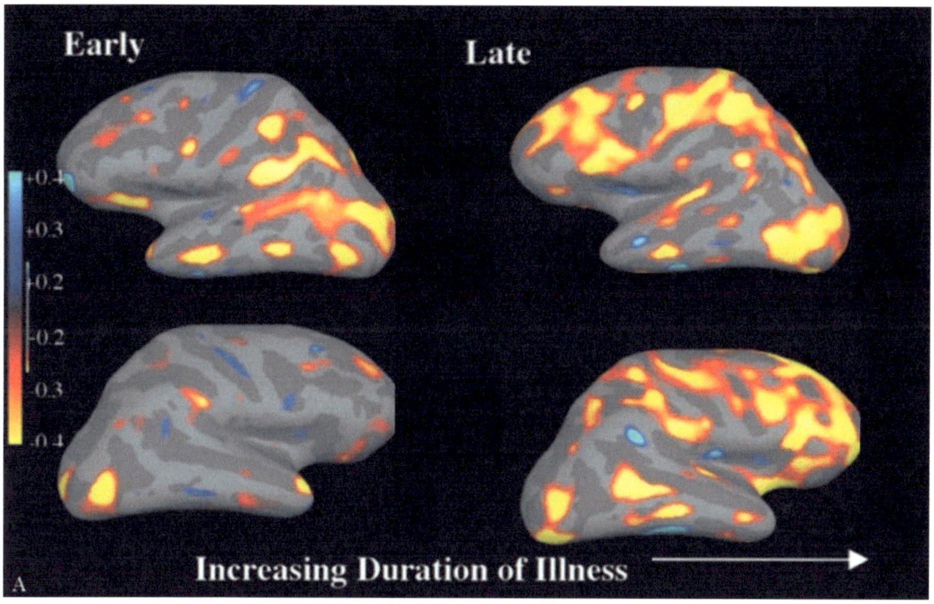

Figure 2.
(A) Mean thickness maps. The surface reconstruction demonstrates mean thickness differences of three different subjects with Huntington's disease (HD) in differing stages of the disease. Darker gray areas correspond to sulci; lighter gray areas correspond to gyri [52].

loss' prognostic value for manifest HD conversion is less evident, with inconsistent findings in two large observational investigations [48, 69]. White matter atrophy, on the other hand, does track disease progression and is present from the earliest premanifest stage through established disease.

2.3.2 Functional MRI

There is mounting evidence that the severity of clinical manifestations in HD is influenced not just by neuronal loss but also by neuronal dysfunction and circuitry rearrangement, and that these processes can occur early in the disease, possibly even before neurodegeneration. By monitoring the hemodynamic response (blood flow) of neural activation, functional neuroimaging methods such as functional MRI (fMRI) produce dynamic images of the brain that aid in elucidating neural activity. Data from manifest HD patients revealed decreased task-activation in multiple subcortical and cortical regions, as well as increased task-activation in various cortical areas, which was interpreted as a compensatory mechanism for task performance [70–75]. Interestingly, premanifest HD gene carriers who were further away from illness onset showed increased activation in multiple brain regions, whereas premanifest HD gene carriers who were closer to disease onset showed lower activation in the striatum [76–79].

Both premanifest and manifest HD gene carriers have exhibited intrinsic deficits in functional connectivity in resting-state fMRI data [80–82]. Reduced blood-oxygen-level-dependent (BOLD) synchronization between the caudate and premotor cortex was reported in premanifest HD gene carriers [80]. A study found several abnormal networks in both premanifest and manifest HD subjects using a method that measures changes in synchrony in BOLD signal amplitude and across space.

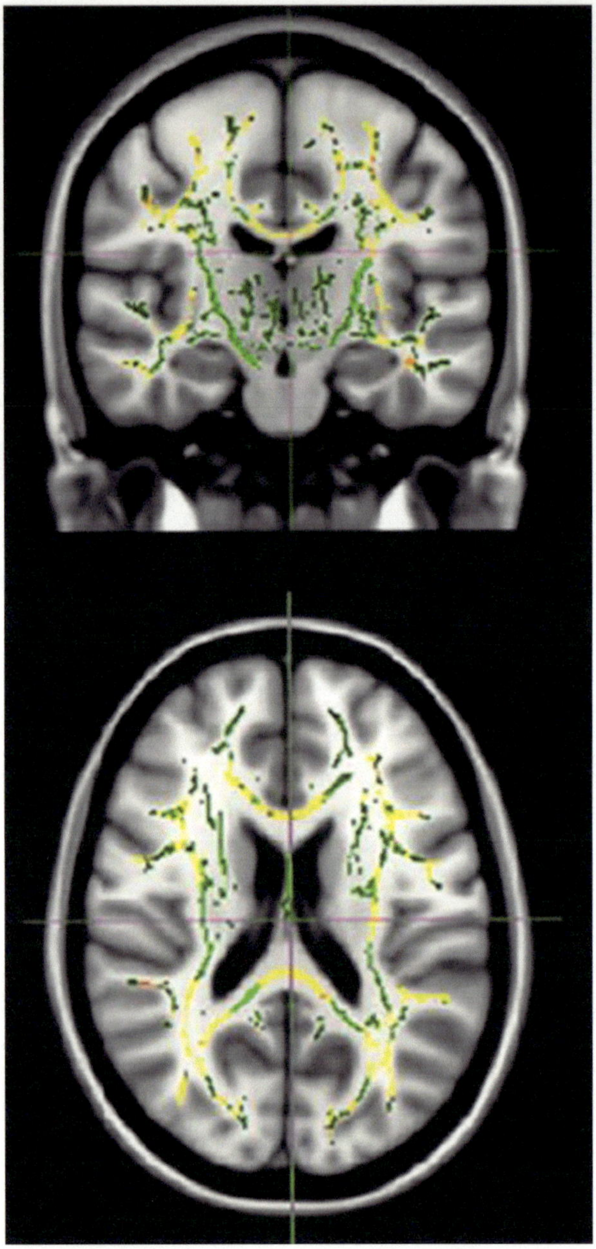

Figure 3.
Tracts showing lower fractional anisotropy in Huntington's disease gene carriers when compared with controls. Results (red-yellow [lower to higher statistical values]) are projected on a white matter skeleton (green), overlaid on a customized mean fractional anisotropy image [58].

For example, it has been found that premanifest HD gene carriers had lower resting-state synchronization in the sensory-motor network and that this level of synchrony was related to motor performance as determined by speeded self-paced tapping [83]. Overall, these data demonstrate aberrant functional network connection in both premanifest and manifest HD, implying that resting state fMRI could be valuable for detecting early neural dysfunction and tracking disease progression.

Premanifest HD gene carriers have also been discovered to have neurovascular changes. Cortical arteriolar cerebral blood volume (CBVa) was significantly elevated in premanifest HD gene carriers compared to normal controls, which was connected with genetic parameters including the CAG-age product score and estimated years to onset [84].

2.3.3 Diffusion MRI

Diffusion MRI assesses the microstructural integrity of white matter filaments, providing additional information to volumetric MRI. The diffusion of water in different directions within the brain is measured using this technique. Water diffusion in healthy white matter fibers is usually only in one direction, making them anisotropic. When white matter breaks down, for example, due to axonal injury or demyelination, diffusion increases in directions other than the axons. Diffusion MRI might, in theory, reveal neuronal injury or dysfunction that occurs before volumetric loss.

The most widely-studied diffusion technique in HD is diffusion tensor imaging (DTI). Across various neurodegenerative diseases, reductions in fractional anisotropy (FA) and increases in mean diffusivity (MD) are commonly observed [85–87] indicating their sensitivity but lack of specificity to the underlying neurodegenerative process. Axonal loss, demyelination, and less cohesive white matter tracts are thought to be the cause of these abnormalities, which would be expected to occur before volume loss.

A Diffusion metric change has been observed in premanifest HD in cross-sectional investigations, particularly in the corpus callosum, internal capsule, and thalamic radiations [88–91]. These alterations in the white matter, particularly the frontal, parietal, and occipital white matter, become increasingly pronounced and extensive in manifest HD [92–94]. The results of longitudinal studies using diffusion metrics have proved inconclusive. Two studies in premanifest HD failed to find 12–30 month changes [89, 95], whereas two larger studies found progressive changes over 1–5 years in premanifest HD cohorts including those up to 10 years away from onset [90, 96]. In manifest-HD, longitudinal alterations in DTI measures have also been demonstrated [51].

Changes in regional DTI measurements have been linked to total motor score (TMS), timed finger tapping, executive function [80], apathy [97], and depression [98]. However, no research has looked into the effectiveness of DTI measurements in predicting clinical development. Furthermore, DTI measurements had smaller impact sizes than volumetric measures in a comparative investigation across periods of 6–15 months [99] limiting the use of DTI as a biomarker of HD progression.

Recent advances in diffusion acquisition and modeling techniques, such as the use of neurite orientation dispersion and density imaging (NODDI) methods (**Figure 4**), have the potential to improve the sensitivity of diffusion MRI measures in HD [100–102]. However, there is currently a lack of agreement on diffusion imaging acquisition parameters, processing, and analysis procedures, which accounts for some of the variance in findings to date.

2.3.4 Positron emission tomography (PET)

The use of PET in the diagnosis and understanding of neurological pathologies is crucial. It is a non-invasive molecular imaging technology that uses

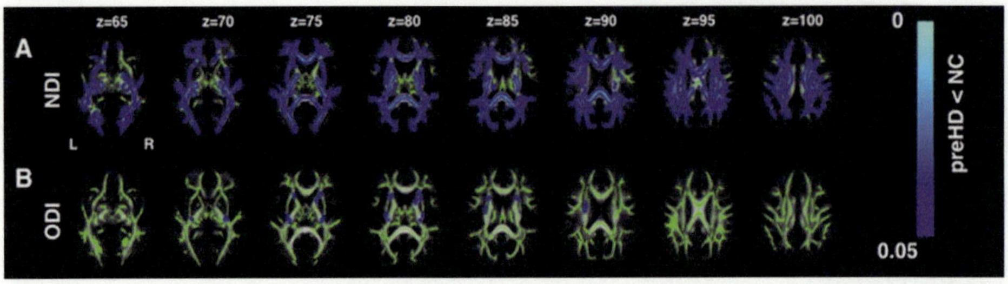

Figure 4.
White matter abnormalities: Neurite orientation dispersion and density imaging (NODDI) analysis [100].

radiopharmaceuticals to attach to a specific molecular target, such as a transporter or receptor, after crossing the blood–brain barrier, allowing accurate tracking of changes in their function. PET now has a wide range of radiolabeled biomarkers for neuroimaging in psychiatry and neurodegenerative diseases like Parkinson's disease (PD), Alzheimer's disease (AD), and Huntington's disease (HD).

PET has been used in HD to investigate metabolic markers of hypo-metabolism, dopaminergic function, microglial activation, and the expression of the PDE10A enzyme [103]. However, similar research have been conducted in small numbers, with mixed results. PET scanning is also more expensive than volumetric or diffusion MRI, generally is less available for large multicenter studies, and is more invasive because it uses ionizing radiation. PET, on the other hand, has the advantage of being able to provide more detailed information about pathological processes, and a future use of PET as a biomarker for target engagement in smaller proof-of-concept or phase 1 trials is in the horizon. PET was recently used to demonstrate effective target engagement of a new PDE10A inhibitor after a single dosage, paving the way for continued clinical development into a phase 2 trial [104]. Amyloid PET has shown promise in both experimental and clinical studies of Alzheimer's disease [105] and a ligand capable of binding a pathogenic form of mutant huntingtin protein could be a useful PET biomarker for relevant pathology and regional brain tissue target engagement in huntingtin lowering studies [106].

3. Artificial intelligence and machine-learning techniques

Computational methods such as machine learning techniques are very useful tools in helping and improving the diagnosis as well as the disease monitoring process. A recent review study [107] concentrated on artificial intelligence in neurodegenerative diseases such as Huntington's disease and others in which the authors reviewed the available tools with focus on machine learning techniques. Many authors have concentrated on Huntington's disease alone using artificial intelligence and machine learning techniques [108–110]. More details on using artificial intelligence and machine learning techniques in the diagnosis and monitoring of Huntington's disease will be reviewed alone later in a future publication.

4. Conclusion

As Huntington's disease is not a preventable or curative disease, the availability of a diagnostic, prognostic, or response biomarker will have significant importance either in premanifest or manifest stage. Reliable biomarkers are needed either to delay/prevent the appearance of symptoms, slow the progression of the disease, and/or to monitor response to the therapy.

The identification of imaging and other measurements that have the ability to monitor and predict disease progression and therapy response has recently progressed in HD biomarker research. The most promising of them appear to be suitable for providing target engagement and efficacy readouts in premanifest HD or at short intervals. Such biomarkers may be verified as surrogate endpoints or even in the clinical context to guide prognostic discussions and treatment decisions in HD in the future as viable medicines become available. This promise will be realized through ongoing efforts to standardize methodology and reproduce findings in large-scale cohorts.

Conflict of interest

The authors declare no conflict of interest.

Author details

Omar Deeb[1]*, Afnan Atallah[2] and Sawsan Salameh[1]

1 Faculty of Pharmacy, Al-Quds University, Jerusalem, Palestine

2 Faculty of Medicine, Al-Quds University, Jerusalem, Palestine

*Address all correspondence to: deeb.omar@gmail.com

References

[1] Killoran A. Biomarkers for Huntington's disease: A brief overview. Journal of Rare Diseases Research and Treatment. 2016;**1**(2):46-50

[2] Unified Huntington's Disease Rating Scale. Reliability and consistency. Huntington Study Group. Moving Disord. 1996;**11**(2):136-142

[3] Zeun P, Scahill RI, Tabrizi SJ, Wild EJ. Fluid and imaging biomarkers for Huntington's disease. Molecular and Cellular Neurosciences. 2019;**97**:67-80

[4] Tabrizi SJ, Scahill RI, Durr A, Roos RA, Leavitt BR, Jones R, et al. Biological and clinical changes in premanifest and early stage Huntington's disease in the TRACK-HD study: The 12-month longitudinal analysis. Lancet Neurology. 2011;**10**(1):31-42

[5] Paulsen JS, Hayden MR, Stout JC, Langbehn DR, Aylward EH, Ross CA, et al. Preparing for preventive clinical trials: The predict-HD study. Archives of Neurology. 2006;**63**(6):883-890

[6] Biomarkers and Surrogate Endpoints. Preferred definitions and conceptual framework. Clinical Pharmacology and Therapeutics. 2001;**69**(3):89-95

[7] Group F-NBW. BEST (Biomarkers, EndpointS, and other Tools) Resource [Internet]. Food and Drug Administration (US); 2016 [cited 2022 Jan 7]. Available from: https://www.ncbi.nlm.nih.gov/books/NBK326791/

[8] Silajdžić E, Björkqvist M. A critical evaluation of wet biomarkers for Huntington's disease: Current status and ways forward. Journal of Huntingtons Diseases. 2018;**7**(2):109-135

[9] Tabrizi SJ, Langbehn DR, Leavitt BR, Roos RAC, Durr A, Craufurd D, et al. Biological and clinical manifestations of Huntington's disease in the longitudinal TRACK-HD study: Cross-sectional analysis of baseline data. Lancet Neurology. 2009;**8**(9):791-801

[10] Bechtel N, Scahill RI, Rosas HD, Acharya T, van den Bogaard SJA, Jauffret C, et al. Tapping linked to function and structure in premanifest and symptomatic Huntington disease. Neurology. 2010;**75**(24):2150-2160

[11] Paulsen JS, Smith MM, Long JD. PREDICT HD investigators and Coordinators of the Huntington Study Group. Cognitive decline in prodromal Huntington Disease: Implications for clinical trials. Journal of Neurology, Neurosurgery, and Psychiatry. 2013;**84**(11):1233-1239

[12] Björkqvist M, Wild EJ, Thiele J, Silvestroni A, Andre R, Lahiri N, et al. A novel pathogenic pathway of immune activation detectable before clinical onset in Huntington's disease. The Journal of Experimental Medicine. 2008;**205**(8):1869-1877

[13] Mochel F, Charles P, Seguin F, Barritault J, Coussieu C, Perin L, et al. Early energy deficit in Huntington Disease: Identification of a plasma biomarker traceable during disease progression. PLoS One. 2007;**2**(7):e647

[14] Byrne LM, Wild EJ. Cerebrospinal fluid biomarkers for Huntington's disease. Journal of Huntingtons Disease. 2016;**5**(1):1-13

[15] Wild EJ, Boggio R, Langbehn D, Robertson N, Haider S, Miller JRC, et al. Quantification of mutant

huntingtin protein in cerebrospinal fluid from Huntington's disease patients. The Journal of Clinical Investigation. 2015;**125**(5):1979-1986

[16] Rodrigues FB, Byrne LM, McColgan P, Robertson N, Tabrizi SJ, Zetterberg H, et al. Cerebrospinal fluid inflammatory biomarkers reflect clinical severity in Huntington's disease. PLoS One. 2016;**11**(9):e0163479

[17] Rodrigues FB, Byrne LM, Tortelli R, Johnson EB, Wijeratne PA, Arridge M, et al. Mutant huntingtin and neurofilament light have distinct longitudinal dynamics in Huntington's disease. Science Translational Medicine. 2020;**12**(574):eabc2888

[18] Johnson EB, Byrne LM, Gregory S, Rodrigues FB, Blennow K, Durr A, et al. Neurofilament light protein in blood predicts regional atrophy in Huntington disease. Neurology. 2018;**90**(8):e717-e723

[19] Byrne LM, Rodrigues FB, Blennow K, Durr A, Leavitt BR, Roos RAC, et al. Neurofilament light protein in blood as a potential biomarker of neurodegeneration in Huntington's disease: A retrospective cohort analysis. Lancet Neurology. 2017;**16**(8):601-609

[20] Rodrigues FB, Byrne L, McColgan P, Robertson N, Tabrizi SJ, Leavitt BR, et al. Cerebrospinal fluid total tau concentration predicts clinical phenotype in Huntington's disease. Journal of Neurochemistry. 2016;**139**(1):22-25

[21] Dalrymple A, Wild EJ, Joubert R, Sathasivam K, Björkqvist M, Petersén Å, et al. Proteomic profiling of plasma in Huntington's disease reveals neuroinflammatory activation and biomarker candidates. Journal of Proteome Research. 2007;**6**(7):2833-2840

[22] Gruber B, Kłaczkow G, Jaworska M, Krzysztoń-Russjan J, Anuszewska EL, Zielonka D, et al. Huntington' disease--imbalance of amino acid levels in plasma of patients and mutation carriers. Annals of Agricultural and Environmental Medicine. 2013;**20**(4):779-783

[23] Wang R, Ross CA, Cai H, Cong W-N, Daimon CM, Carlson OD, et al. Metabolic and hormonal signatures in pre-manifest and manifest Huntington's disease patients. Frontiers in Physiology. 2014;**23**(5):231

[24] Leoni V, Caccia C. The impairment of cholesterol metabolism in Huntington disease. Biochimica et Biophysica Acta. 2015;**1851**(8):1095-1105

[25] Leoni V, Mariotti C, Nanetti L, Salvatore E, Squitieri F, Bentivoglio AR, et al. Whole body cholesterol metabolism is impaired in Huntington's disease. Neuroscience Letters. 2011;**494**(3):245-249

[26] Lazar AS, Panin F, Goodman AOG, Lazic SE, Lazar ZI, Mason SL, et al. Sleep deficits but no metabolic deficits in premanifest huntington's disease. Annals of Neurology. 2015;**78**(4):630-648

[27] Danielle M B. Neuroendocrine and neurotrophic signaling in Huntington's disease: Implications for pathogenic mechanisms and treatment strategies | Elsevier Enhanced Reader [Internet]. [cited 2022 Jan 5]. Available from: https://reader.elsevier.com/reader/sd/pii/S0149763416302767?token=8AC86ED510FC2DF4BF8B1DF8056A8CFF9E2D9E7FB7EA133A1663311A9ED49B9DED3F68B270B5BD69AB338543DB0D0144&originRegion=eu-west-1&originCreation=20220105192925

[28] Block RC, Dorsey ER, Beck CA, Brenna JT, Shoulson I. Altered cholesterol and fatty acid metabolism in Huntington

disease. Journal of Clinical Lipidology. 2010;**4**(1):17-23

[29] Herzog-Krzywoszanska R, Krzywoszanski L. Sleep disorders in Huntington's disease. Frontiers in Psychiatry. 2019;**12**(10):221

[30] Videnovic A, Lazar AS, Barker RA, Overeem S. The clocks that time us'—Circadian rhythms in neurodegenerative disorders. Nature Reviews Neurology. 2014;**10**(12):683-693

[31] Browne SE, Ferrante RJ, Beal MF. Oxidative stress in Huntington's disease. Brain Pathology. 1999;**9**(1):147-163

[32] Johri A, Beal MF. Antioxidants in Huntington's disease. Biochimica et Biophysica Acta. 2012;**1822**(5):664-674

[33] Trushina E, McMurray CT. Oxidative stress and mitochondrial dysfunction in neurodegenerative diseases. Neuroscience. 2007;**145**(4):1233-1248

[34] Sayre LM, Perry G, Smith MA. Oxidative stress and neurotoxicity. Chemical Research in Toxicology. 2008;**21**(1):172-188

[35] Sandyk R. The endogenous opioid system in neurological disorders of the basal ganglia. Life Sciences. 1985;**37**(18):1655-1663

[36] Niemela V, Landtblom A-M, Nyholm D, Kneider M, Constantinescu R, Paucar M, et al. Proenkephalin decreases in cerebrospinal fluid with symptom progression of Huntington's disease. Movement Disorders. 2021;**36**(2):481-491

[37] Al Shweiki MR, Oeckl P, Pachollek A, Steinacker P, Barschke P, Halbgebauer S, et al. Cerebrospinal fluid levels of prodynorphin-derived peptides are decreased in Huntington's disease. Movement Disorders. 2021; **36**(2):492-497

[38] Dong X, Cong S. MicroRNAs in Huntington's disease: Diagnostic biomarkers or therapeutic agents? Frontiers in Cellular Neuroscience. 2021;**15**:705348

[39] Langfelder P, Gao F, Wang N, Howland D, Kwak S, Vogt TF, et al. MicroRNA signatures of endogenous Huntingtin CAG repeat expansion in mice. PLoS One. 2018;**13**(1):e0190550

[40] Ananbeh H, Vodicka P, Kupcova SH. Emerging roles of exosomes in Huntington's disease. International Journal of Molecular Sciences. 2021;**22**(8):4085

[41] Liu W, Bai X, Zhang A, Huang J, Xu S, Zhang J. Role of exosomes in central nervous system diseases. Frontiers in Molecular Neuroscience [Internet]. 2019 [cited 2022 Feb 1];12. Available from: https://www.frontiersin.org/article/10.3389/fnmol.2019.00240

[42] Zhang X, Abels ER, Redzic JS, Margulis J, Finkbeiner S, Breakefield XO. Potential transfer of polyglutamine and CAG-repeat RNA in extracellular vesicles in Huntington's disease: Background and evaluation in cell culture. Cellular and Molecular Neurobiology. 2016;**36**(3):459-470

[43] Johnson EB, Gregory S, Johnson HJ, Durr A, Leavitt BR, Roos RA, et al. Recommendations for the use of automated gray matter segmentation tools: Evidence from Huntington's disease. Frontiers in Neurology. 2017;**8**:519

[44] Wijeratne PA, Garbarino S, Gregory S, Johnson EB, Scahill RI, Paulsen JS, et al. Revealing the timeline of structural MRI changes in premanifest

to manifest Huntington disease. Neurology Genetics. Oct 2021;7(5):e617

[45] Aylward EH, Sparks BF, Field KM, Yallapragada V, Shpritz BD, Rosenblatt A, et al. Onset and rate of striatal atrophy in preclinical Huntington disease. Neurology. 2004;**63**(1):66-72

[46] Tabrizi SJ, Reilmann R, Roos RAC, Durr A, Leavitt B, Owen G, et al. Potential endpoints for clinical trials in premanifest and early Huntington's disease in the TRACK-HD study: Analysis of 24 month observational data. Lancet Neurology. 2012;**11**(1):42-53

[47] Aylward EH, Nopoulos PC, Ross CA, Langbehn DR, Pierson RK, Mills JA, et al. Longitudinal change in regional brain volumes in prodromal Huntington disease. Journal of Neurology, Neurosurgery, and Psychiatry. 2011;**82**(4):405-410

[48] Tabrizi SJ, Scahill RI, Owen G, Durr A, Leavitt BR, Roos RA, et al. Predictors of phenotypic progression and disease onset in premanifest and early-stage Huntington's disease in the TRACK-HD study: Analysis of 36-month observational data. Lancet Neurology. 2013;**12**(7):637-649

[49] Rosas HD, Liu AK, Hersch S, Glessner M, Ferrante RJ, Salat DH, et al. Regional and progressive thinning of the cortical ribbon in Huntington's disease. Neurology. 2002;**58**(5):695-701

[50] Rosas HD, Salat DH, Lee SY, Zaleta AK, Pappu V, Fischl B, et al. Cerebral cortex and the clinical expression of Huntington's disease: Complexity and heterogeneity. Brain. 2008;**131**(Pt 4):1057-1068

[51] Gregory S, Cole JH, Farmer RE, Rees EM, Roos RAC, Sprengelmeyer R, et al. Longitudinal diffusion tensor imaging shows progressive changes in white matter in Huntington's disease. Journal of Huntingtons Diseases. 2015;**4**(4):333-346

[52] Crawford HE, Hobbs NZ, Keogh R, Langbehn DR, Frost C, Johnson H, et al. Corpus callosal atrophy in premanifest and early Huntington's disease. Journal of Huntingtons Diseases. 2013;**2**(4):517-526

[53] Johnson EB, Ziegler G, Penny W, Rees G, Tabrizi SJ, Scahill RI, et al. Dynamics of cortical degeneration over a decade in Huntington's disease. Biological Psychiatry. 2021;**89**(8):807-816

[54] Fischl B, Sereno MI, Tootell RB, Dale AM. High-resolution intersubject averaging and a coordinate system for the cortical surface. Human Brain Mapping. 1999;**8**(4):272-284

[55] Dale AM, Fischl B, Sereno MI. Cortical surface-based analysis. I. Segmentation and surface reconstruction. Neuroimage. 1999;**9**(2): 179-194

[56] Brodmann K. Vergleichende Lokalisationslehre der Grosshirnrinde in ihren Prinzipien dargestellt auf Grund des Zellenbaues [Internet]. Leipzig : Barth; 1909 [cited 2022 Jan 13]. 346 p. Available from: http://archive.org/details/b28062449

[57] Squitieri F, Cannella M, Simonelli M, Sassone J, Martino T, Venditti E, et al. Distinct brain volume changes correlating with clinical stage, disease progression rate, mutation size, and age at onset prediction as early biomarkers of brain atrophy in Huntington's disease. CNS Neuroscience & Therapeutics. 2009;**15**(1):1-11

[58] Dierks T, Linden DE, Hertel A, Günther T, Lanfermann H, Niesen A, et al. Multimodal imaging of residual function and compensatory resource

allocation in cortical atrophy: A case study of parietal lobe function in a patient with Huntington's disease. Psychiatry Research. 1999;**90**(1):67-75

[59] Paulsen JS, Nopoulos PC, Aylward E, Ross CA, Johnson H, Magnotta VA, et al. Striatal and white matter predictors of estimated diagnosis for Huntington disease. Brain Research Bulletin. 2010;**82**(3-4):201-207

[60] Aylward EH, Anderson NB, Bylsma FW, Wagster MV, Barta PE, Sherr M, et al. Frontal lobe volume in patients with Huntington's disease. Neurology. 1998;**50**(1):252-258

[61] Halliday GM, McRitchie DA, Macdonald V, Double KL, Trent RJ, McCusker E. Regional specificity of brain atrophy in Huntington's disease. Experimental Neurology. 1998;**154**(2):663-672

[62] Rosas HD, Koroshetz WJ, Chen YI, Skeuse C, Vangel M, Cudkowicz ME, et al. Evidence for more widespread cerebral pathology in early HD: An MRI-based morphometric analysis. Neurology. 2003;**60**(10):1615-1620

[63] Beglinger LJ, Nopoulos PC, Jorge RE, Langbehn DR, Mikos AE, Moser DJ, et al. White matter volume and cognitive dysfunction in early Huntington's disease. Cognitive and Behavioral Neurology. 2005;**18**(2):102-107

[64] Jech R, Klempír J, Vymazal J, Zidovská J, Klempírová O, Růzicka E, et al. Variation of selective gray and white matter atrophy in Huntington's disease. Movement Disorders. 2007;**22**(12):1783-1789

[65] Scahill RI, Hobbs NZ, Say MJ, Bechtel N, Henley SMD, Hyare H, et al. Clinical impairment in premanifest and early Huntington's disease is associated with regionally specific atrophy. Human Brain Mapping. 2013;**34**(3):519-529

[66] Beckman KB, Ames BN. Oxidative decay of DNA. The Journal of Biological Chemistry. 1997;**272**(32):19633-19636

[67] Della Nave R, Ginestroni A, Tessa C, Giannelli M, Piacentini S, Filippi M, et al. Regional distribution and clinical correlates of white matter structural damage in Huntington disease: A tract-based spatial statistics study. AJNR. American Journal of Neuroradiology. 2010;**31**(9):1675-1681

[68] Rosas HD, Reuter M, Doros G, Lee SY, Triggs T, Malarick K, et al. A tale of two factors: What determines the rate of progression in Huntington's disease? A longitudinal MRI study. Moving Disorders. 2011;**26**(9):1691-1697

[69] Gregory S, Johnson E, Byrne LM, Rodrigues FB, Henderson A, Moss J, et al. Characterizing white matter in Huntington's disease. Moving Disorders in Clinical Practise. 2020;**7**(1):52-60

[70] Clark VP, Lai S, Deckel AW. Altered functional MRI responses in Huntington's disease. Neuroreport. 2002;**13**(5):703-706

[71] Kim J-S, Reading SAJ, Brashers-Krug T, Calhoun VD, Ross CA, Pearlson GD. Functional MRI study of a serial reaction time task in Huntington's disease. Psychiatry Research. 2004;**131**(1):23-30

[72] Georgiou-Karistianis N, Sritharan A, Farrow M, Cunnington R, Stout J, Bradshaw J, et al. Increased cortical recruitment in Huntington's disease using a Simon task. Neuropsychologia. 2007;**45**(8):1791-1800

[73] Georgiou-Karistianis N, Stout JC, Domínguez DJF, Carron SP,

Ando A, Churchyard A, et al. Functional magnetic resonance imaging of working memory in Huntington's disease: Cross-sectional data from the IMAGE-HD study. Human Brain Mapping. 2014;**35**(5):1847-1864

[74] Thiruvady DR, Georgiou-Karistianis N, Egan GF, Ray S, Sritharan A, Farrow M, et al. Functional connectivity of the prefrontal cortex in Huntington's disease. Journal of Neurology, Neurosurgery, and Psychiatry. 2007;**78**(2):127-133

[75] Paulsen JS, Zimbelman JL, Hinton SC, Langbehn DR, Leveroni CL, Benjamin ML, et al. fMRI biomarker of early neuronal dysfunction in presymptomatic Huntington's Disease. AJNR. American Journal of Neuroradiology. 2004;**25**(10):1715-1721

[76] Wolf RC, Vasic N, Schönfeldt-Lecuona C, Landwehrmeyer GB, Ecker D. Dorsolateral prefrontal cortex dysfunction in presymptomatic Huntington's disease: Evidence from event-related fMRI. Brain. 2007;**130** (Pt 11):2845-2857

[77] Reading SAJ, Dziorny AC, Peroutka LA, Schreiber M, Gourley LM, Yallapragada V, et al. Functional brain changes in presymptomatic Huntington's disease. Annals of Neurology. 2004;**55**(6):879-883

[78] Wolf RC, Sambataro F, Vasic N, Schönfeldt-Lecuona C, Ecker D, Landwehrmeyer B. Aberrant connectivity of lateral prefrontal networks in presymptomatic Huntington's disease. Experimental Neurology. 2008;**213**(1):137-144

[79] Dumas EM, van den Bogaard SJA, Hart EP, Soeter RP, van Buchem MA, van der Grond J, et al. Reduced functional brain connectivity prior to and after disease onset in Huntington's disease. Neuroimage Clinic. 2013;**2**:377-384

[80] Poudel GR, Egan GF, Churchyard A, Chua P, Stout JC, Georgiou-Karistianis N. Abnormal synchrony of resting state networks in premanifest and symptomatic Huntington disease: The IMAGE-HD study. Journal of Psychiatry & Neuroscience. 2014;**39**(2):87-96

[81] Werner CJ, Dogan I, Saß C, Mirzazade S, Schiefer J, Shah NJ, et al. Altered resting-state connectivity in Huntington's disease. Human Brain Mapping. 2014;**35**(6):2582-2593

[82] Unschuld PG, Joel SE, Liu X, Shanahan M, Margolis RL, Biglan KM, et al. Impaired cortico-striatal functional connectivity in prodromal Huntington's Disease. Neuroscience Letters. 2012;**514**(2):204-209

[83] Hua J, Unschuld PG, Margolis RL, van Zijl PCM, Ross CA. Elevated arteriolar cerebral blood volume in prodromal Huntington's disease. Movement Disorders. 2014;**29**(3): 396-401

[84] Zhang Y, Schuff N, Du A-T, Rosen HJ, Kramer JH, Gorno-Tempini ML, et al. White matter damage in frontotemporal dementia and Alzheimer's disease measured by diffusion MRI. Brain. 2009;**132**(Pt 9):2579-2592

[85] Atkinson-Clement C, Pinto S, Eusebio A, Coulon O. Diffusion tensor imaging in Parkinson's disease: Review and meta-analysis. Neuroimage Clinic. 2017;**16**:98-110

[86] Slattery CF, Zhang J, Paterson RW, Foulkes AJM, Carton A, Macpherson K, et al. ApoE influences regional white-matter axonal density loss in Alzheimer's disease. Neurobiology of Aging. 2017;**57**:8-17

[87] Rosas HD, Lee SY, Bender AC, Zaleta AK, Vangel M, Yu P, et al. Altered white matter microstructure in the corpus callosum in Huntington's disease: Implications for cortical "disconnection.". NeuroImage. 2010;**49**(4):2995-3004

[88] Stoffers D, Sheldon S, Kuperman JM, Goldstein J, Corey-Bloom J, Aron AR. Contrasting gray and white matter changes in preclinical Huntington disease: An MRI study. Neurology. 2010;**74**(15):1208-1216

[89] Poudel GR, Stout JC, Domínguez DJF, Salmon L, Churchyard A, Chua P, et al. White matter connectivity reflects clinical and cognitive status in Huntington's disease. Neurobiology of Disease. 2014;**65**:180-187

[90] Harrington DL, Long JD, Durgerian S, Mourany L, Koenig K, Bonner-Jackson A, et al. Cross-sectional and longitudinal multimodal structural imaging in prodromal Huntington's disease. Movement Disorders. 2016;**31**(11):1664-1675

[91] Rosas HD, Tuch DS, Hevelone ND, Zaleta AK, Vangel M, Hersch SM, et al. Diffusion tensor imaging in presymptomatic and early Huntington's disease: Selective white matter pathology and its relationship to clinical measures. Movement Disorders. 2006;**21**(9):1317-1325

[92] Bohanna I, Georgiou-Karistianis N, Egan GF. Connectivity-based segmentation of the striatum in Huntington's disease: Vulnerability of motor pathways. Neurobiology of Disease. 2011;**42**(3):475-481

[93] Bonneh-Barkay D, Bissel SJ, Kofler J, Starkey A, Wang G, Wiley CA. Astrocyte and macrophage regulation of YKL-40 expression and cellular response in neuroinflammation. Brain Pathology. 2012;**22**(4):530-546

[94] Hobbs NZ, Cole JH, Farmer RE, Rees EM, Crawford HE, Malone IB, et al. Evaluation of multi-modal, multi-site neuroimaging measures in Huntington's disease: Baseline results from the PADDINGTON study. Neuroimage Clin. 2012;**2**:204-211

[95] Odish OFF, Leemans A, Reijntjes RHAM, van den Bogaard SJA, Dumas EM, Wolterbeek R, et al. Microstructural brain abnormalities in Huntington's disease: A two-year follow-up. Human Brain Mapping. 2015;**36**(6):2061-2074

[96] Shaffer JJ, Ghayoor A, Long JD, Kim RE-Y, Lourens S, O'Donnell LJ, et al. Longitudinal diffusion changes in prodromal and early HD: Evidence of white-matter tract deterioration. Human Brain Mapping. 2017;**38**(3):1460-1477

[97] Delmaire C, Dumas EM, Sharman MA, van den Bogaard SJA, Valabregue R, Jauffret C, et al. The structural correlates of functional deficits in early huntington's disease. Human Brain Mapping. 2013;**34**(9):2141-2153

[98] Sprengelmeyer R, Orth M, Müller H-P, Wolf RC, Grön G, Depping MS, et al. The neuroanatomy of subthreshold depressive symptoms in Huntington's disease: A combined diffusion tensor imaging (DTI) and voxel-based morphometry (VBM) study. Psychological Medicine. 2014;**44**(9):1867-1878

[99] Hobbs NZ, Farmer RE, Rees EM, Cole JH, Haider S, Malone IB, et al. Short-interval observational data to

inform clinical trial design in Huntington's disease. Journal of Neurology, Neurosurgery, and Psychiatry. 2015;**86**(12):1291-1298

[100] Kaden E, Kelm ND, Carson RP, Does MD, Alexander DC. Multi-compartment microscopic diffusion imaging. NeuroImage. 2016;**139**:346-359

[101] Zhang J, Gregory S, Scahill RI, Durr A, Thomas DL, Lehericy S, et al. In vivo characterization of white matter pathology in premanifest huntington's disease. Annals of Neurology. 2018;**84**(4):497-504

[102] Zhang H, Schneider T, Wheeler-Kingshott CA, Alexander DC. NODDI: Practical in vivo neurite orientation dispersion and density imaging of the human brain. NeuroImage. 2012;**61**(4):1000-1016

[103] Wilson H, De Micco R, Niccolini F, Politis M. Molecular imaging markers to track Huntington's disease pathology. Frontiers in Neurology. 2017;**8**:11

[104] Delnomdedieu M, Forsberg A, Ogden A, Fazio P, Yu C-R, Stenkrona P, et al. In vivo measurement of PDE10A enzyme occupancy by positron emission tomography (PET) following single oral dose administration of PF-02545920 in healthy male subjects. Neuropharmacology. 2017;**117**:171-181

[105] Laforce R, Soucy J-P, Sellami L, Dallaire-Théroux C, Brunet F, Bergeron D, et al. Molecular imaging in dementia: Past, present, and future. Alzheimer's & Dementia. 2018;**14**(11):1522-1552

[106] MacDonald D, Borrowsky B, Bard J, Cachope R, Park L, Wityak J, et al. Dominguez and T. Vogt. Pharmacodynamic Biomarkers for HTT-Lowering Therapies. 2015

[107] Tăuțan AM, Ionescu B, Santarnecchi E. Artificial intelligence in neurodegenerative diseases: A review of available tools with a focus on machine learning techniques. Artificial Intelligence in Medicine. 2021;**117**:102081. DOI: 10.1016/j.artmed.2021.102081

[108] Gaßner H, Jensen D, Marxreiter F, Kletsch A, Bohlen S, Schubert R, et al. Gait variability as digital biomarker of disease severity in Huntington's disease. Journal of Neurology. Jun 2020;**267**(6):1594-1601. DOI: 10.1007/s00415-020-09725-3. Epub 2020 Feb 11. 2020 Mar 27;: PMID: 32048014; PMCID: PMC7293689

[109] Odish OFF, Johnsen K, van Someren P, Roos RAC, van Dijk JG. EEG may serve as a biomarker in Huntington's disease using machine learning automatic classification. Scientific Reports. 2018;**8**(1):16090

[110] Xiang C, Cong S, Liang B, Cong S. Bioinformatic gene analysis for potential therapeutic targets of Huntington's disease in pre-symptomatic and symptomatic stage. Journal of Translational Medicine. 2020;**18**(1):388

Chapter 4

Neuroimaging Biomarkers for Huntington's Disease

Nadine van de Zande, Eidrees Ghariq, Jeroen de Bresser and Susanne de Bot

Abstract

Biomarkers are of great importance in the prediction of onset and follow-up of patients with Huntington's disease (HD). Neuroimaging is a convenient biomarker, because of its non-invasive character. Since technology is continuously evolving, we are increasingly able to visualize detailed neural structures and functions. Furthermore, it could also identify new targets for therapeutic interventions. In this chapter, we review findings in neuroimaging research applied to HD. First, we will describe the neuroanatomical structures and cellular processes, which are important in the pathophysiology of HD and are therefore particularly interesting to focus on. We will then discuss the different imaging modalities; from structural to functional, from commonly used to novel imaging strategies. Striatal- and cortical-volume loss on conventional MRI and decrease in uptake of radiotracers on PET are currently the most robust markers of disease progression. The use of other MRI-metabolites, specific PET radioligands, DTI, and fMRI may have the potential to detect HD pathology earlier and more accurately but needs further investigation. These neuroimaging markers, possibly combined, can be useful clinical outcome measures in clinical trials and could improve the management and treatment of future patients.

Keywords: neuroimaging, biomarkers, Huntington's disease, MRI, fMRI, PET

1. Introduction

Huntington's disease (HD) is an autosomal dominant inherited neurodegenerative disorder caused by an expansion of a CAG repeat in the huntingtin gene. Therefore, confirmation of carrier ship of an expanded CAG repeat is achieved by a genetic test, which can be performed years before disease onset [1]. The clinical diagnosis and follow-up of the disease are obtained by standardized clinical scales like the Unified Huntington's Disease Rating Scale (UHDRS) [2]. This assessment consists of a specific neurological exam (e.g. 'Total Motor Score', TMS), Total Functional Capacity (TFC), and neuropsychological assessments. During the neuropsychological assessments cognitive, psychological, and psychiatric information is obtained. Clinical diagnosis in research and in clinic is grounded on a clinician's rating of the diagnostic confidence level. The clinical diagnosis requires a level of 4, on a 0–4 scale, completely based on the motor features of HD. Although these assessments are standardized

 IntechOpen

and well-known, they have their limitations. In particular, the subjective nature of these assessments contributes to a high inter-rater variability [3]. They also show low sensitivity to longitudinal change and monitoring of treatment effects [4]. There are often many observable clinical and functional changes before motor onset. Since the clinical diagnosis is not made until motor symptoms appear, there is a large gray area where symptoms already exist without being officially classified as 'manifest'.

At this moment, there is no successful disease-modifying therapy for HD. Nevertheless, research trials are constantly evolving, hoping to find solutions in the near future. Sensitive biomarkers are of great importance in these clinical trials. These are valuable not only for accurate group selection, or deciding when to start therapy, but are also important for evaluating treatment response, which is currently measured by the earlier mentioned clinical scales. The Biomarkers Definitions Working Group defines a biomarker as 'a characteristic that is objectively measured and evaluated as an indicator of normal biological processes, pathogenic processes, or pharmacologic responses to a therapeutic intervention' [5]. A biomarker must be widely available, reliable, reproducible and it should show low variability in the normal population. Besides that, it has to change in relation to disease progression and disease-modifying treatment. An ideal biomarker should be able to predict disease onset and should be obtained in a minimally invasive manner.

Neuroimaging biomarkers are convenient, as they are relatively non-invasive and can provide an accurate picture of the pathophysiology. Currently, there are different types of neuroimaging methods, sequences, and tools available and many of them have been used in observational studies of patients with HD. In this chapter, we summarize the results of different neuroimaging modalities that have been used in HD research. Furthermore, we will discuss the qualities and the limitations of these modalities and appraise which type of methods we should favor for future clinical trials. Before moving to a discussion of the neuroimaging modalities, we first elaborate on the pathophysiology of HD to determine the relevant neuroanatomical structures and cellular processes that neuroimaging modalities should focus on.

2. From neuropathology to scan

HD is a neurodegenerative disease caused by CAG repeat expansion in the huntingtin gene (HTT) on chromosome 4. The number of CAG repeats is associated with an increased accumulation of abnormal huntingtin protein in the neurons. When the CAG-repeat rises above a threshold of 36 repeats, this leads to cumulative toxicity [1]. The CAP score, a statistical prediction tool developed by Penney and colleagues, is an index to *estimate* the degree of cumulative exposure to the effects of the CAG repeat expansion. The score considers the length of repeats and the lifetime exposure to the disease burden. It can be used to predict the clinical status of HD expanded gene carriers (HDEGC), as it has proven to be a good predictor of HD pathology in post-mortem brains [6]. In general, it is believed that the longer the CAG repeat, the earlier the age of disease onset [7]. However, CAG repeat length is certainly not the only predictor of clinical outcome, as similar CAG repeat lengths can lead to many different manifestations of the disease (e.g. variable age of onset) [8].

An important part of the pathology of HD is the accumulation of mutant huntingtin protein to form intranuclear inclusions, which subsequently leads to loss of GABAergic medium spiny neurons (MSNs) in the neostriatum [9, 10]. This includes the caudate nucleus and the putamen, but also other regions of the basal ganglia, such as the globus pallidus. Multiple studies have shown this striatal atrophy, making it the hallmark of HD's pathology [11, 12]. Degeneration of inhibitory MSNs leads to hyperactivity of the dopaminergic pathway, contributing to chorea [13]. As the pathology progresses, neuronal degeneration spreads to the cortex and other extrastriatal regions [12, 14, 15]. All four cerebral lobes undergo cortical thinning with a layer-specific neuronal loss [16]. Cerebellar symptoms are quite common in HD, including dysarthria and ataxic movements of extremities. Although less studied, recent studies also show a reduction of the cerebellar volume [17]. Considering all these findings, HD is now being viewed as a multisystemic disease [16]. Further research in this area is needed. There is no current explanation why these cortical and subcortical brain regions are selectively affected, ultimately leading to HD-specific neurodegeneration.

Disease-specific cellular processes can be investigated using neuroimaging techniques like magnetic resonance spectroscopy (MRS), iron sensitive MRI, and PET-scans. The loss of post-synaptic striatal MSNs results in a decline of post-synaptic dopaminergic neurons. Phosphodiesterase (PDE) is an enzyme that seems to play a role in the pathophysiology of HD. This is an intracellular enzyme that plays an important role in cell signal transduction and in promoting neuronal survival. PDE10A is predominantly expressed in the striatum and has an essential role in regulating dopaminergic signaling. In mutated HD models, it has been shown that mutant huntingtin decreases striatal PDE10A expression [18] and a decreased PDE10A level has been identified before onset of symptoms [19].

Besides the dopaminergic receptors, there are several other receptors suggested to be involved in HD pathophysiology. One of them is the GABA receptor. Studies have shown a decreased GABA receptor density in the caudate, putamen, and the frontal cortex in post-mortem HD brains [20]. In the globus pallidus an increased level of GABA receptors was found [21]. Another common receptor that seems to play a role in HD pathophysiology is the adenosine type 1 receptor, which plays a role in neuroprotection and autoregulation of cerebral blood flow [22]. Cannabinoid type 1 receptors (CB1R) are expressed in the basal ganglia, predominantly in the GABAergic striatal MSNs. They seem to be important for motor and cognitive function and play a protective role against excitotoxicity and promote neuronal survival [23, 24]. Transgenic HD mouse models showed decreased levels of CB1R [25] in both premanifest and manifest stages, with a further decline during the manifest stages [26].

Iron accumulation [27], synaptic dysfunction [28, 29] as well as mitochondrial dysfunction [30] are other mechanisms of HD pathophysiology. Iron accumulation has been correlated with aging and increased accumulation has been found in several neurodegenerative diseases like HD [27]. It is currently unknown whether iron accumulation is a cause or a consequence of neurodegeneration. Iron accumulates in microglia, as has been shown in HD [31]. Microglia cells are also involved in neuroinflammation, another probable pathological process in HD. Activated microglia cells have a neuroprotective effect, but overactivation can result in neuronal damage due to toxic levels of free radicals, nitric oxide and interleukins. Activated microglia have been found in the neostriatum, globus pallidus, cortex, and subcortical white matter in post-mortem human brain tissue in HDEGC [32]. It remains unclear whether this activation is a compensatory mechanism in response to the loss of neurons, or whether microglia activation itself is the cause of pathophysiology.

3. Magnetic resonance imaging

Magnetic Resonance Imaging (MRI) is an imaging method where a magnetic field, magnetic gradients and radiofrequency pulses are used to change the state of hydrogen atoms in the brain. These changes create energy which is subsequently measured and exported in the form of an MR image [33].

There are different approaches in methodology when analyzing a scan. There is a region-of-interest (ROI) approach and a whole-brain analysis approach. The first one is driven by known pathologically affected structures, the latter is more exploratory, unbiased and does not require a priori assumptions. ROI studies can be useful to study specific hypotheses since they often show high sensitivity for detecting differences between groups and demonstrating longitudinal change. The delineation of ROIs can be performed manually or by using automated software. Although manual delineation of ROIs is the gold standard, it is very time consuming and is susceptible to inter- and intra-rater variability. The automated software can define ROIs on a more consistent level across studies and is therefore likely to be used more frequently in future studies. However, there is an increased level of error to include some of the surrounding tissue in the analysis while working with these automated software methods. ROI approaches are used in volumetric imaging as well as diffusion-weighted imaging (DWI) [34].

Whole-brain-analysis enables exploratory analysis across all brain regions. It has been widely used in HD studies, for example, to measure brain volume. Voxel-based morphometry (VBM) is the most commonly used approach. With this approach volumetric differences in the gray matter, white matter, and cerebrospinal fluid (CSF) can be measured between different groups. It can also be used to make associations between volume and other biomarkers [35]. Cortical thickness is another whole-brain approach, widely used in HD studies. In DWI a whole-brain analysis can be performed by using Tract-Based Spatial Statistics (TBSS). This compares diffusion metrics across the brain. Another type of analysis that is used in DWI is tractography. This is used to measure diffusivity between two or more regions of interest [36].

3.1 Volumetric MRI

Structural or volumetric MRI scans can be used to measure anatomical features of the brain, such as volume and cortical thickness. They are usually 3D T1 weighted sequences, after which volume measurements are made using software packages [37]. Each body tissue has a different relaxation time that is dependent on how tightly bound the protons are in their environment. Volumetric MRI studies were the first and are still the most common in vivo imaging studies in HD research.

MRI-based brain volume measurements have been introduced in HD at the beginning of the 1990s. The most common finding is striatal atrophy. Harris et al. were the first to discover a volume loss in the putamen and caudate, comparing 15 symptomatic HDEGC with 19 healthy controls [38]. In 1996, they were able to discriminate manifest HDEGC from healthy controls using volume measurements [39]. In the early years of structural MRI research, Aylward et al. did multiple studies showing that striatal atrophy was already present years before clinical motor diagnosis [40–42]. Contemporary scientists have confirmed these findings, showing volume loss up to 24 years before clinical motor onset [43–45].

Longitudinal studies show reducing striatal volumes with decreasing time to estimated diagnosis, with striatal volumes markedly reduced compared to age-matched controls at the time of clinical motor diagnosis [46–48]. In the past years there have been four large multicentre studies, aimed at identifying sensitive and reliable biomarkers. TRACK-HD is one of these studies, following 120 premanifest and 123 early manifest HDEGC longitudinally [43, 49, 50]. After a 12-month follow-up, they measured a mean volume loss of 1.4% and 2.9% in the caudate, and 2.3% and 4.5% in the putamen, compared with baseline for the premanifest and manifest HDGC group, respectively [49]. After a 24-month follow-up, this atrophy progressed in both groups [4]. IMAGE-HD, another multicentre longitudinal study, showed that longitudinal volume change in the caudate was the only measure among a range of multi-modal imaging features that discriminated between groups across different disease stages (e.g. >15 years from clinical motor onset, <15 years from clinical motor onset, and after clinical motor onset). Caudate volume showed statistically bigger longitudinal change than putamen volume, over 30 months [51]. This larger difference in caudate volume loss compared to putamen atrophy was confirmed by another multicentre study called PADDINGTON [48].

While striatal atrophy can already be detected years before onset, cortical atrophy becomes more apparent after clinical motor diagnosis [52–54]. Atrophy in the frontal lobe has been identified in the moderate and late stages of HD. Volume reductions have been identified in almost all brain structures, including the total cerebrum, cerebral cortex, basal ganglia, amygdala, hippocampus, brainstem, and cerebellum [52, 53]. Another study showed an association between increased losses of gray matter volume in the occipital, parietal, frontal and insular cortices, and disease progression [55]. However, in the TRACK-HD study whole brain and gray matter atrophy were already found in premanifest HDEGC with <10.8 years from predicted symptomatic onset. In the premanifest HD group >10.8 years from predicted symptomatic onset atrophy was limited to the striatum, the white matter surrounding the striatum, the corpus callosum, and the posterior white matter tract [50]. Volume loss in total brain matter and white matter progressed after a 12-month follow-up [49]. The fourth large longitudinal multicentre study, PREDICT-HD, showed volume loss in total brain, white matter, cortical gray matter, thalamus, caudate, and putamen volume in premanifest HDEGC when compared to controls. Striatal volume, especially the putamen, showed the largest loss of volume [46, 47, 56]. White matter atrophy has been identified in more studies, showing volume loss early in the disease, continuing to decline with disease progression [43, 44, 48, 49, 54]. One recent imaging study using both PET and MRI, found significant volume loss in caudate, putamen, and pallidum in premanifest HDEGC. In the early manifest HDEGC, they also found significant atrophy in the thalamus, occipital and frontal cortex, and whole gray matter [57].

Cortical thinning has also been found in early manifest HD, affecting the sensorimotor areas, the occipital, and prefrontal cortices [58–60]. Thinning of the cortical gray matter can be detected before clinical diagnosis, becoming more pronounced and proceeding from posterior to anterior regions as the disease progresses [43, 53, 59, 60].

There is overwhelming evidence showing associations between brain volume loss and clinical outcome measures, showing a decline in performance with reducing volumes. Striatal atrophy has been associated with predicted time to clinical disease onset, age of onset, disease duration, and an increasing CAP score [40, 47, 61]. After a 36-month follow-up, the TRACK-HD study showed progressive whole brain, caudate, putamen, and gray matter atrophy in early manifest HDEGC which correlated to a decreasing TFC score. In the premanifest group with >10.8 years from predicted motor onset, striatal atrophy was not associated with a decline in motor and cognitive performances [50]. This was confirmed by a recent multimodal imaging study, where they also found significant striatal atrophy in premanifest HDEGC which did not correlate to clinical measures [62]. In the TRACK-HD study, the premanifest group within 10.8 years from predicted motor onset did show a significant decline of motor and cognitive performances. Besides this, TRACK-HD showed that striatal and gray volume measures were sensitive predictors of conversion from the premanifest to manifest HD stage [50]. Furthermore, at the most advanced disease stage ($7 \leq \text{TFC} \leq 10$) the caudate volume showed a constant rate of decline over the 12-, 24-, and 36-month follow-up periods. Whole-brain and caudate volumetric MRI measurements have a substantially better power analysis than standard clinical outcome measures used in current clinical trials (TMS and TFC). They only need one-sixth of the sample size to detect the same degree of slowing [63]. The PADDINGTON study, which looked at longitudinal changes in early manifest HDEGC compared to healthy controls, found more MRI changes than changes in clinical outcome measures [64].

In premanifest HDEGC and early HD manifest patients subtle impairments were correlated with regional brain volume, especially in the caudate, putamen, and globus pallidus [65–67]. Regional cortical atrophy has also been correlated with MMSE, TFC, and motor scores [52, 60]. Regional cortical thinning was found to be correlated with cognitive decline [68, 69], depression [69], and TMS [70]. Atrophy in the precentral and parieto-occipital regions correlated with TFC, clinical motor, and cognitive scores [71–73]. Associations have been found between atrophy in the caudate and worse outcome scores on the mini-mental state examination (MMSE) [39], TMS, SDMT, and TFC [74]. A voxel-based morphometry showed an inverse correlation between the TMS and the concentrations of caudate nuclei tissue, internal capsule, occipital lobes, cerebellum, lower brainstem (corrected for age and CAG repeat length) [75]. Increased atrophy in the putamen also correlates with motor impairment [38, 39]. Thalamic atrophy was found to be associated with apathy [76]. Atrophy in the thalamus, insula and white matter volume has been associated with cognitive performance scores in both pre-manifest and manifest HD groups [77, 78].

It can be concluded that volume loss occurs many years before the development of motor signs that mark the clinical diagnosis of HD, starting with striatal atrophy and concomitantly spread over the gray and white matter. To study the microstructural changes that could explain neuronal loss and to find approaches for disease-modifying treatments, other imaging modalities are necessary.

3.2 Diffusion tensor imaging

DWI is a newer MRI technique that has been extensively used in HD research for the past two decades. It is based upon the diffusion properties of protons in the intra- and extracellular space. In an unrestricted space, water molecules can move in any direction, which is called isotropic movement. When the path of the water molecules is restricted, such as along a white matter tract, water diffuses in an anisotropic way. Diffusion tensor imaging (DTI) is a specific type of DWI that enables a more precise assessment of the direction of diffusion. DTI allows measurement of the orientation, strength, and directionality of the diffusion of water molecules. The measures that can be derived from DTI are mean diffusivity (MD), fractional anisotropy (FA), axial diffusivity (AD), and radial diffusivity (RD). MD represents the speed of diffusion, where a low MD value represents a restricted diffusion and a high MD value an unrestricted diffusion (e.g., CSF). FA represents the strength of the main direction of diffusion. FA values range from 0 to 1. When the FA value is close to 0 there is an equal diffusion in all directions, as is the case in CSF. AD is the diffusion rate along the main axis of diffusion and an increase in AD reflects axonal degeneration and loss. RD is the rate of diffusion in the transverse direction, where an increase in RD reflects the demyelination of white matter tracts [79].

The advantage of DTI is that it can detect microstructural changes, which precedes the larger changes that appear on a volumetric MRI image [80]. This applies especially to the white matter, due to the white matter tracts.

As with structural MRI, diffusion imaging has been used in large multicentre imaging trials like TRACK-HD, TRACK-ON HD, PADDINGTON, IMAGE-HD, and PREDICT-HD. These large MRI datasets are important to improve the technical standardization and statistical power of clinical DTI studies in HD.

Widespread diffusion abnormalities have been demonstrated in both manifest and premanifest HDEGC [81]. Multiple studies have shown a decreased FA and increased AD, RD, and MD in a wide range of white matter regions for HDEGC compared to healthy controls [82–91]. Among these studies three of them included symptomatic HDEGC and healthy controls [87, 89, 91] and three studies compared premanifest HDEGC and controls [83, 84, 90]. There have been many more studies showing a decrease in FA, of which Reading and colleagues were the very first. They showed lower FA values in the precentral cortex of premanifest HDEGC [92]. The TRACK-ON HD study, a longitudinal study of 72 premanifest HDEGC over 24 months, identified that cortico-striatal connections were most affected, followed by interhemispheric and intrahemispheric connections [93]. The corpus callosum has been studied frequently in DTI-studies, probably due to its easy access and well-organized pattern of the pathway. In 2010, Rosas et al. found an increase in AD and RD in fibers of the corpus callosum for the first time, suggesting a cortical disconnection between the prefrontal cortical regions [94]. Also the basal ganglia, the surrounding white matter tracts between these regions and the cortex have been analyzed thoroughly using DTI. There have been studies looking at both white matter and gray matter, showing an increase of FA in the gray matter and a decrease of FA in the white matter for HD patients compared to controls [95–103]. Other studies showed that diffusion imaging could be used as a method to differentiate the subgroup close-to-onset premanifest HDEGC from far-from-onset HDEGC. They showed an increased MD in close-to-onset-HD, compared to far-from-onset and healthy controls [104, 105].

There are also studies with contradictory results. Syka and colleagues did not find any significant difference between FA and MD in the pallidum of symptomatic HDEGC compared to healthy control [106]. Poudel et al. and Matsui et al. have found increased RD without a difference in AD in HDEGC, suggestive of myeline pathology [107, 108].

The longitudinal IMAGE-HD study showed a progressive increase in MD located in the caudate, putamen and corpus callosum of premanifest HDEGC after 18 and 30 months follow-up [51, 109]. Sampedro and colleagues studied 39 HDEGC in different stages and showed correlations between MD and disease progression [110]. Other longitudinal diffusion studies did find cross-sectional differences, but did not find significant longitudinal effects in the included groups [70, 88, 111–113].

Diffusion studies have also tried to correlate diffusion to different phenotypes, clinical signs and genetic variables. Changes in diffusion have been linked to increased impairment in neuropsychological performance [69, 70, 98] and motor assessments [69, 70, 114]. For example, Bohanna et al. showed a positive correlation between motor symptoms and an increase in diffusion in the corpus callosum [91]. Philips and colleagues showed correlations between diffusion and clinical and genetic variables, such as CAG and cognitive assessments [115]. Microstructural dissociation in WM tracts has been associated with depression [69], apathy [116], and irritability [117]. Combining both volumetric and diffusion data sets, Georgiou-Karistianis and his group could accurately detect individuals up to 15 years before onset of symptoms, making it a valuable biomarker [118].

In summary, it seems that MD is increased in widespread regions of the brain and FA is reduced in white matter regions when comparing HDEGC to controls. This difference already begins in the premanifest phase of the disease and increases with disease progression. These results indicate an important role in white matter disorganization in HD.

3.3 Magnetic resonance spectroscopy

MRS is an MRI technique that can look on a microscopic level at the pathophysiology. It uses protons, like hydrogen protons, to measure metabolite concentrations. This modality does not give structural information about the brain tissue, but enables an interpretation of the chemical composition of the tissue. The most common metabolites are N-acetylaspertate (NAA), which is a marker for neuronal and axonal integrity; creatine, reflecting brain energy metabolism; choline, a glial marker; glutamate, a neurotransmitter; lactate, a product of anaerobic glycolysis; and myo-inositol, an astrocyte marker [119]. To date, no previous studies have shown a pathognomic alteration of any metabolite for HD [120]. In manifest HDEGC lower NAA and creatine have been measured in the putamen and/or caudate nucleus [121–125] and thalamus [126]. Adanyeguh et al. found a significantly higher total creatine in the visual cortex and a significantly lower total creatine in the striatum, in manifest HDEGC compared to controls [127]. This decreased level of total creatine has also been found in premanifest HDEGC in some studies [121, 125], of which one was part of the multicentred TRACK-HD study [121]. Other studies did not show a decreased level in premanifest HDEGC [128, 129]. MRS studies looking at glutamate levels in HDEGC did not demonstrate consistent results either. Some of these studies found increased levels of glutamate [130–132], others found no difference with healthy controls [121, 122] or found a lower level compared to controls [121, 127]. Choline was found to be decreased in the frontal cortex of premanifest HDEGC [128] and the NAA/choline ratio was found to be decreased in the frontal cortex of manifest HDEGC [133]. Furthermore, increased myo-inositol was measured in the putamen of manifest HDEGC [121] and increased lactate has been assessed in the basal ganglia, cerebellum and occipital, parietal, and frontal cortex of manifest HDEGC [123, 124, 133, 134]. Correlations have been made between alternations in metabolites and motor performance [121, 125], neuropsychological performance [128], disease severity [133], and disease burden [121]. So far there have been two longitudinal MRS studies, both showing no longitudinal change of metabolites in their follow-up [135, 136].

3.4 Iron sensitive MRI

Various MRI techniques have been used, trying to assess iron accumulation. One of these techniques is the use of relaxation rates R2 and R2* when using the T2 and T2* sequences, respectively. This susceptibility measurement cannot distinguish between paramagnetic or diamagnetic entities and therefore cannot conclude whether there is iron or myeline pathology or calcifications. Susceptibility weighted imaging (SWI) is another widely applied method to visualize iron deposition, although it is not able to provide quantitative measures. One of the more novel techniques to measure magnetic susceptibility is quantified susceptibility mapping (QSM). This technique can differentiate between diamagnetic and paramagnetic and can quantify the iron measures.

Multiple studies have shown increased iron levels in the basal ganglia in early manifest HDEGC compared to controls [137–143]. Some studies also found a decreased level of iron deposition in the frontal white matter [137, 140], parieto-occipital cortex [144], and in the substantia nigra and hippocampus. More novel studies have also included premanifest HDEGC, often showing an increased iron level in the caudate [145], putamen, and globus pallidus [146] as well [142–144, 147]. One study from Sanchez-Castaneda et al. showed an increased iron level in the caudate, staying relatively stable throughout disease progression, whereas iron levels in the putamen and globus pallidus increased progressively [144]. Iron-sensitive MRI studies have found correlations between iron levels and CAG repeat [139, 140, 144, 145, 147], increasing disease severity [138, 139, 141, 142, 144] and were found to be independent of volume [138].

4. Functional MRI

Functional MRI (fMRI) is an imaging technique that measures brain activity by using changes in blood oxygenation due to hemodynamic (blood flow) response to neuronal activity (Blood Oxygen Level-Dependent [BOLD]). This BOLD signal represents the ratio between oxygenated and deoxygenated blood and can be used as a measure of local neural activity. fMRI can be obtained in a resting state (rs-fMRI), where you can analyze the function between interacting regions, focusing on network connectivity or connectomics. Task-Based fMRI is another way to measure neural function connectivity, by doing a particular task or function while being in the MRI-scanner. It investigates the neurovascular response to these tasks [148].

Like in structural MRI there are different ways to investigate the neural activity. Task-based fMRI is usually done on a voxel-by-voxel basis. With rs-fMRI you can use seed-based analyses or independent component analysis. Seed-based analysis is partly hypothesis-driven and looks at a predefined region, compared to the rest of the brain. Independent component analysis is not based on predefined knowledge. Functional connectomics can be made by using both these rs-fMRI methods [149]. Current studies often correct functional connectivity for loss of volume.

Functional activity is highly dependent on the type of task and the region of the brain that is analyzed. Furthermore, when applying task-based fMRI in a multicentre imaging trial, this can entail a higher degree of variability in the performed tasks. Therefore, comparing fMRI studies and interpreting them can be very difficult [81].

4.1 Resting state-fMRI

rs-fMRI studies have been used to examine functional networks in HD populations. They overcome the variability in task performances that come along with task-based fMRI. In recent years, there is an increase in studies looking at the entire connectome. Studies using a seed-based analysis often look at functional networks like known motor and cognitive networks. They also regularly include the default mode network (DMN), a network that becomes active when the brain is at rest. These studies show reduced connectivity in the DMN of HDEGC compared to controls, suggesting a disrupted connection when the brain is at rest [150, 151]. Reduced connectivity in manifest HDEGC has been found within the basal ganglia, between the basal ganglia and the insula and between the primary motor cortex and the insula [97]. Also, premanifest HDEGC has shown reduced connectivity within the primary motor cortex [152], between the premotor cortex and the caudate nucleus [153], and in the somatosensory cortex [154]. This reduced connectivity in both premanifest and manifest HDEGC correlated with motor performance [97, 152, 154]. Another study showed reduced connectivity between the cerebellum and the paracentral gyrus, which correlated with disease burden and motor signs [155]. Reduced connectivity in the lower fusiform gyrus, which is important in the visual network, correlated with disease burden and symbol digit modality test (SDMT) scores [156]. Functional connectivity was also found to be reduced in the dorsal attention network in both premanifest and manifest HD, correlating with cognitive decline [154].

Studies investigating functional connectivity in the executive network found both reduced [151, 156] and increased connectivity [154, 156, 157] in manifest HD. This difference in connectivity seems to follow different spatial trajectories: parietal cortex and subcortical structures get a decreased connectivity in manifest stages' [151, 154, 156], while increased connectivity is measured in the frontal cortex [156–158]. McColgan et al. confirmed this difference in connection per region using connectomics [159]. Increased connectivity was also found in the supplementary motor area (SMA) and motor cortex, correlating with worsening of motor performance, in manifest HD patients [156, 157, 160]. Other regions with increased connectivity in manifest HDEGC were bilateral caudate, inferior and middle frontal cortices [156], striatum, thalamus, and frontal regions [157]. Increased CAG repeat length correlated with increasing fronto-occipital connectivity and decreasing connectivity within the visual cortex [161]. A recent rs-fMRI study, using a 7 T MRI-scanner, found functional connectivity to be decreased between the premotor cortex and the striatum as well as between the SMA and the premotor cortex in both premanifest and manifest HDEGC compared to controls. The connectivity was increased between the striatum and both the frontal inferior and frontal middle region. They also found a significant correlation between the TMS and the connectivity in the premotor regions and between the UDHRS behavioral score and the connectivity in the frontal middle regions. The CAP score and estimated years to onset correlated with functional dysconnectivity between the striatum and frontal region, and between the premotor cortex and the SMA, suggesting a potentially valuable biomarker [162]. Some rs-fMRI studies show an association between increased frontal connectivity and more preserved cognitive function [163, 164], suggesting a compensatory response.

Some studies have also shown a difference in disconnection between premanifest and manifest expanded gene carriers. While reduced connectivity was found between frontal and motor cortex and within the medial visual network for both premanifest and manifest HDEGC, reduced connectivity in the deep gray matter and occipital cortex was only detected in manifest HDEGC [151]. Other studies have found no difference in the functional connectivity of the visual network between premanifest HDEGC and healthy controls [60, 165]. Coppen and colleagues did find a significant decrease in functional connectivity in this area in the manifest patients [60].

So far, studies have not found a longitudinal change in connectivity [165–167]. One study did a follow-up of a premanifest HDEGC cohort and found no change in connectivity after 3 years [165].

4.2 Task-based fMRI

Multiple task-based fMRI studies have shown changes in activation in manifest HD patients compared to controls, correcting for brain atrophy [168–171]. Something that has been identified more than once is a hyperactivation in certain regions in premanifest HDEGC, while other regions show a decreased activation. In one study they found a decreased activation in the posterior cingulate and hyperactivation in the left anterior prefrontal cortex in premanifest HDEGC [160]. Klöppel et al. found increased activation in the supplementary motor area (SMA) after a finger tapping task in premanifest HDEGC, especially in the HDEGC subgroup closest to onset [172]. They also found increased activation in the right parietal cortex in response to a working memory task, with a correlation to atrophy [164]. This increased activation suggests compensation in the premanifest phase of the disease. Other studies in premanifest HDEGCs confirmed this hyperactivation. In premanifest HDEGC *far-from-onset* hyperactivation was found in the left sensorimotor cortex [173], anterior cingulate and preSMA [174], and subcortical structures [175]. In only one study, hypoactivity was found in the anterior cingulate in premanifest HDEGC *far-from-onset* [173]. In the premanifest subgroup *close-to-onset* hypoactivation was found in the subcortical structures [174, 175], SMA, left insula, right inferior frontal gyrus [173], and dorsolateral prefrontal cortex [176]. Besides Klöppel et al. [172], one other study found hyperactivation in premanifest HDEGC *close-to-onset*, in the left inferior parietal and right superior frontal regions [176]. The multimodal study of Pini et al., where they used volumetric MRI, DTI, and fMRI, confirmed these differences in premanifest HDEGC subgroups. In *far-from-onset* premanifest HDEGC, there was increased connectivity in the left caudate-cortical functional pathway compared to the healthy controls. No significant differences were found between the *close-to-onset* subgroup and healthy controls. There was also no difference between the total premanifest group and controls with regard to functional connectivity of the right caudate nucleus, bilateral putamen, and bilateral nucleus accumbens [105]. These differences in activity and locations sometimes differ from each other, partly due to differences in task designs. Therefore, no real conclusion can be made about the exact time point in the premanifest phase when and the brain region where hyperactivation takes place. However, it's quite clear that there is regional increased activation somewhere during the premanifest phase of the disease, possibly far-from-onset. This is often interpreted as compensation for dysfunctional circuits elsewhere [177].

Several longitudinal fMRI studies have shown none or little evidence of longitudinal changes in activity. Dominguez et al. followed 29 controls, 35 premanifest HDEGC, and 18 manifest HDEGC and showed no changes in activity in either the controls or the premanifest HDEGC after a period of 30 months. The symptomatic HDEGC did show a reduction over time [168]. Poudel and colleagues showed no longitudinal change in activation in early manifest HDEGC and controls after a follow-up of 30 months [178]. However, in the premanifest cohort, there was a progressive increase in activation in the dorsolateral prefrontal cortex and frontal regions over 18 months [179] and over 30 months [178]. Also, Wolf et al. found no evidence of longitudinal changes in activity after a 2-year follow-up of 13 premanifest HDEGC and 13 controls [180].

There have been fMRI studies that relate neural activity to specific symptoms, especially neuropsychiatric symptoms [154]. One study found a positive correlation between depressive symptoms and activation of the ventromedial prefrontal cortex during the Stroop interference task, in premanifest HDEGC [153]. This correlation was more significant with longer CAG repeats. Gray et al. found an association between reduced prefrontal activation in symptomatic HDEGC and severe neuropsychiatric problems such as disinhibition and depression [181]. In the longitudinal study of Dominguez and colleagues, the progressive hypoactivation in the right dorsolateral prefrontal cortex and putamen, in symptomatic HDEGC, was found to be associated with disturbances in executive functioning [168].

fMRI studies have shown us that HD is much more than a basal ganglia disorder. It serves as a tool for a better understanding of the underlying pathophysiological mechanisms, especially concerning different symptoms. Task-based fMRI studies have demonstrated compensatory mechanisms, which may serve as an important marker in the premanifest stage before clinical signs develop.

5. PET-scan

PET is a non-invasive molecular imaging technique for the quantitative imaging of biological functions. It involves the injection of a metabolically active compound labeled with a radioactive isotope, also known as radioligand. This radioligand binds to specific targets and emits gamma rays which are detectable by the gamma camera in the PET scanner. Based on the molecular pathophysiology several radioligands have been identified and used in HD imaging studies [182]. These include tracers for cerebral glucose metabolism, postsynaptic dopaminergic receptors, phosphodiesterase (PDE)10A, cannabinoid receptors, GABA receptors, adenosine A1 receptors, presynaptic terminal marker SV2A, and activated microglia as markers of neuroinflammation.

First of all, the most common radioligand is [^{18}F]FDG, which traces the uptake of glucose. Multiple studies using [^{18}F]FDG-PET scans showed glucose hypometabolism in the caudate [73, 183] and putamen [54, 73, 184–186] in manifest HDEGC compared to healthy controls. A decreased glucose metabolism has also been measured in premanifest HDEGC [54, 185, 187]. Some studies have identified hypometabolism in the cortex as well [54, 73, 183, 187]. Researchers have found a progressive decline in glucose metabolism over the years [185, 188] and could correlate decreased metabolism in the caudate [189] and the putamen [190] with predicted time to symptomatic onset. Some of these studies corrected the measured glucose uptake for volumetric loss and found hypometabolism to be independent of atrophy [54, 73, 184, 191]. This makes it plausible that altered glucose metabolism precedes volumetric loss. If metabolism is not corrected for partial volume, metabolic deficits could simply be a consequence of neuronal atrophy. Furthermore, there have been studies correlating hypometabolism with clinical assessments, such as cognitive decline [183, 192] and severity of motor symptoms [186]. A recent study from Sampedro et al., which corrected for partial volume, found frontotemporal hypometabolism which correlated to the severity of apathy, and striatal hypometabolism which correlated with motor and cognitive UHDRS scores [73]. Limitations in FDG-PET studies are the several influencing factors like hyperglycaemia [193] and psychotropic drugs including benzodiazepine which can decrease the (global) brain activity and thus the glucose metabolism [194].

Other radiotracers which are useful in HD research are the ones that trace post-synaptic dopaminergic receptors. D_1 receptors can be investigated using the radioligand [^{11}C]SCH23390 and D_2 receptors are measured by using [^{11}C]raclopride. In PET studies, loss of post-synaptic D_1 and D_2 receptors has been reported in premanifest [195–197] and manifest HDEGC [198, 199]. Longitudinal studies showed an annual loss of striatal D_1 en D_2 receptors and this decline seems to be faster during earlier premanifest disease stages [195, 200]. It has been shown that [^{11}C]raclopride is a more sensitive marker of disease progression than glucose metabolism, showing a higher annual loss of D_2 receptors than a decline of striatal glucose uptake [185]. Furthermore, it has been shown to precede striatal atrophy [201]. Studies have also found correlations between dopaminergic receptor loss and CAG repeat (after correcting for age) [201, 202], severity of cognitive function [203], TMS [204], and TFC [195]. Decreased D_2 binding in the putamen correlated with higher chorea scores on the TMS and cognitive decline [204]. The specific areas *within* the striatum have also been linked to specific clinical manifestations. Motor signs have been linked to loss of dopamine receptors in the sensorimotor striatum [200], while the associative striatum, in addition to the temporal cortex, is more involved in cognitive decline [205]. Cortical reduction in D_2 receptor binding has also been identified in premanifest HDEGC and manifest HDEGC, where the loss of receptors was correlated with worse attention and executive function [205]. Other regions with loss of dopaminergic receptors are the thalamus [203], hypothalamus [206], and frontal and temporal regions [200].

Radioligands that trace PDE10A have been identified in the last decades, such as [^{18}F]MNI-659 and [^{11}C]IMA107. Studies in premanifest [207] and manifest HDEGC show a decrease in PDE10A in the caudate and putamen [208], and also in the globus pallidus [209], compared to healthy controls. Two longitudinal studies showed a progressive decrease in these three regions with disease progression, of which decline in the caudate was the most obvious [210, 211]. Fazio et al. showed a slightly more rapid decline from late premanifest to HD stage I, than from early premanifest to late premanifest. Loss of PDE10A has been correlated with more severe motor scores, disease burden, and striatal atrophy [209]. Several studies have shown that annual changes in PDE10A expression were greater than the annual changes in dopamine D_2 receptors [185, 195, 200, 211]. This makes PDE10A an even more sensitive marker of disease progression than dopaminergic receptors.

Researchers have identified radiotracers that can detect specific receptors that are related to the HD pathophysiology. Van Laere et al. looked at cannabinoid type receptor (CB_1R) levels with the radioligand [^{18}F]MK9470 and found a decreased level in the cortex, brainstem, and cerebellum of early manifest HDEGC. They also found an association between the loss of CB_1R and increased disease burden scores [212]. Ceccarini and colleagues measured CB_1R levels in premanifest HDEGC and found a decreased binding in the prefrontal cortex, which correlated with depression. They included a control group consisting of gene-negative subjects from HD families to control for potential effects of distress caused by growing up in an HD family and undergoing genetic testing [62].

Two PET studies that have looked at GABA receptor expression, using [^{11}C]flumazenil, and glucose uptake, using [^{18}F]FDG, found a lower level of GABA receptors in the caudate of early manifest HDEGC, compared to healthy controls. Glucose uptake was decreased in the caudate, putamen, and thalamus of these HDEGC [213, 214].

One PET study used [^{18}F]CPFPX to look at striatal adenosine A_1 receptors and found a decreased level in the caudate and putamen, in manifest HDEGC compared to healthy controls. There was no significant difference in receptor levels in the caudate and putamen of premanifest HDEGC, compared to healthy controls. However, in the thalamus, they did find a significant increase in A_1 receptor level in premanifest HDEGC far-from-onset, while there was no significant difference in the group close-to-onset [215].

There is one PET-study looking at synaptic damage using the tracer [^{11}C]-UCB-J for the presynaptic terminal marker SV2A. In manifest HDEGC, they found a significant loss of SV2A binding in the putamen, caudate, pallidum, cerebellum and parietal, temporal and frontal cortex, whereas glucose metabolism observed with an ^{18}F-FDG PET was only reduced in the caudate and putamen of these patients. Loss of

SV2A in the putamen correlated with the TMS. In premanifest HDEGC there was only significant decrease in SVA2 in the caudate and putamen [57].

To study the role of neuroinflammation in cerebral and neurodegenerative diseases, radiotracers that bind to activated microglia can be used, e.g. [^{11}C]PK11195. Studies in HD subjects using [^{11}C]PK11195 have shown increased microglial activation in striatal and cortical regions in both premanifest and manifest HDEGC, with a correlation to loss of striatal D_2 receptors [216, 217]. Increased glial activation has also been found in the putamen and pallidum in HDEGC [218]. Studies found microglial activation to be correlated to the severity of motor symptoms [216, 219], disease severity and higher probability of motor onset over the next 5 years [219], and increased levels of interleukins IL-1β, IL-6, IL-8, and TNF-α [220]. Regions of increased activation also seem to differ in disease progression. The dorsal striatum, which is involved in motor and cognitive function, is often affected in premanifest stages. The ventral striatum, involved in psychiatric symptoms, is affected later in the manifest phase [219].

6. Conclusion and future perspectives

Based on the cumulative evidence of the imaging studies included in this chapter, it can be concluded that clinical diagnosis of HD is not the starting point, but rather the endpoint of the neuropathophysiological changes. To summarize the current results of all these neuroimaging modalities along the disease course, we made a hypothetical graph (**Figure 1**). It must be emphasized that this is a hypothetical graph

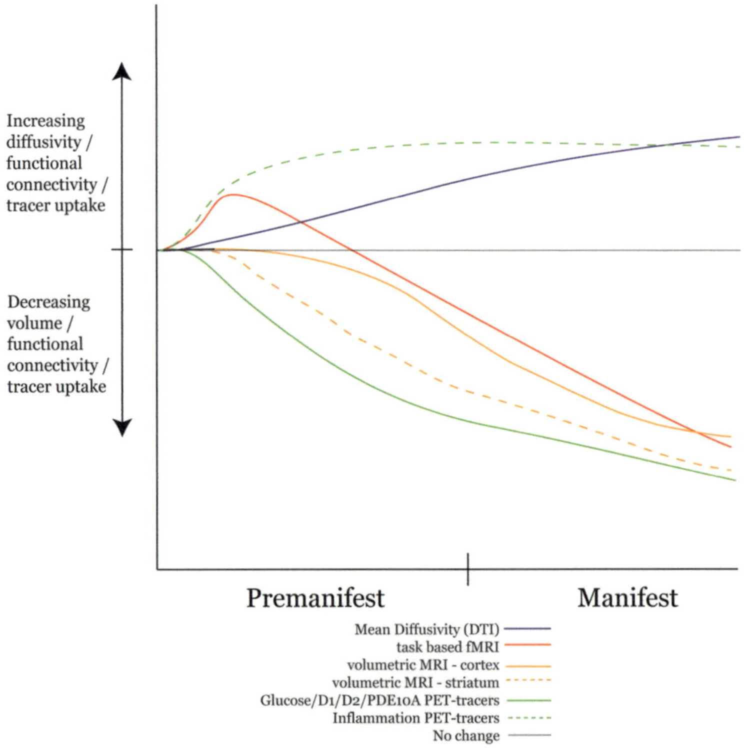

Figure 1.
Course in neuroimaging changes during Huntington's disease progression.

and may change as new studies are published in the future. Certain disease stages, such as the more advanced stages, have not been sufficiently studied with neuroimaging to make any conclusions. Nevertheless, it places current findings in perspective, by comparing the changes for each modality set against disease progression.

MRI-based brain volume measurements have already been used since the beginning of the 1990s in HD research and have consistently identified volume loss in multiple regions of the brain. These volume changes seem to start in the striatum, years before clinical onset and spread over the cortex ending up affecting widespread regions of the gray and white matter. Longitudinal studies have shown decreasing volumes of the striatum and specific cortical regions, which correlated with clinical outcome measures and genetic variables. All these factors make structural MRI a valuable technique that is helpful to predict clinical onset before diagnosis, although it is still not applicable on an individual level.

To analyze the microstructural differences, which develop before volume loss, DTI is a better imaging modality. This especially applies to the analysis of white matter changes. DTI studies have identified diffusion abnormalities in widespread regions of the brain, showing certain areas with decreasing diffusion while others have increasing diffusion measures in the same stage. These ratios seem to correlate with certain genetic and clinical variables. These results suggest a more important role for white matter disorganization in HD than we previously thought. A potential application of this knowledge might be in classifying and understanding HD phenotypes according to the differences observed in diffusion maps. Nevertheless, longitudinal diffusion effects have not been consistently proven to date.

Specific MRI sequences have improved our knowledge of the HD pathophysiology, can be used as a biomarker for stage-conversion, and give insights into alternative approaches for disease-modifying treatments. Iron accumulations and metabolic changes seem to precede clinical diagnosis and progress with advancing disease stages. However, longitudinal data and consistent cross-sectional results are still lacking.

fMRI studies have shown that HD is more than just a basal ganglia disorder, even in the premanifest stages of the disease. Using fMRI studies, we have been able to improve our understanding of the disease's pathophysiology. Increased connectivity after task performance precedes clinical diagnosis, which might be a compensatory mechanism that slows down the conversion into the manifest stage. One of the limitations is that this modality has not been able to consistently detect a significant change over time.

PET-scans can be used to detect early pathophysiological changes before structural changes, like glucose metabolism, neuroinflammation, and receptor level expression. They show a reliable longitudinal effect and correlate with clinical assessments. [^{18}F]FDG PET is a less sensitive marker compared to dopaminergic D2-receptor ligand [^{11}C]raclopride to monitor disease progression. PDE10A expression using different PET-tracers was found to be an even more sensitive marker than dopamine receptor levels. PET-scans improve our knowledge of disease pathophysiology at a molecular level and could help us in evaluating treatment response. At this moment iMagemHTT is in the recruitment phase to study novel mutant huntingtin PET radioligands [^{11}C]CHDI-00485180-R and [^{11}C]CHDI-00485626 and test their suitability for the quantification of aggregated mutant huntingtin in the brain of HDEGC compared to healthy controls [221]. This imaging method combines proteomic knowledge with neuroimaging to improve our knowledge of mHTT aggregation in the brain and it could improve evaluating treatment response.

Multimodal imaging studies, where multiple imaging modalities are used together in one study, are the future of neuroimaging research. To combine these data, researchers have started to use artificial intelligence such as machine learning. It has already been used to develop a multimodality neuroimaging polymarker of HD with the ability to identify HDEGC who are within 5 years of their clinical motor diagnosis. This polymarker consisted of subcortical region volume, cortical thickness, and resting-state functional connectivity [222]. One study used machine learning on neuroimaging datasets to successfully classify between premanifest HDEGC and controls [223]. Mohan et al. recently used machine learning to develop a new disease progression model with nine disease states of increasing severity, based on clinical data only [224]. Another focus in HD-research, requiring artificial intelligence, is the use of network models to explain the pathology of the disease progression and disease phenotypes [158, 225]. However, machine learning algorithms require large amounts of data, before they start to provide useful results, especially when it comes to neural networks. Application in larger imaging studies or the combination of datasets can therefore be expected in the future.

Furthermore, studies should be multicentred to overcome the most common limitation of all included research, which is a small study population. Nevertheless, standardization is not that easy, especially when it concerns advanced MRI-techniques. Despite the excellent performance of different PET-tracers as biomarkers, PET has a major limitation. Not all PET-studies can be performed at every site due to the need for an on-site cyclotron to produce ^{11}C-labeled radioligands.

Using different imaging modalities new pathophysiological mechanisms have been discovered or hypothesized, such as neuroinflammation, iron deposition, cellular reactions, regional deposition of the huntingtin protein. This shines a new light on therapeutic approaches and could serve as a drug target image technique. The imaging of such biomarkers has also some limitations. A biomarker could be relevant only in specific disease stages, after specific physiological events, or present during a limited period of time [5]. An ideal biomarker should change longitudinally, as time and disease progresses. Therefore, longitudinal imaging studies are of great importance. Another characteristic of an ideal biomarker is that it should change in response to disease-modifying treatment, something quite valuable in future clinical trials.

Author details

Nadine van de Zande[1*], Eidrees Ghariq[2,3], Jeroen de Bresser[2] and Susanne de Bot[1]

1 Department of Neurology, Leiden University Medical Centre, Leiden, The Netherlands

2 Department of Radiology, Leiden University Medical Centre, Leiden, The Netherlands

3 Department of Radiology, Medical Spectrum Twente, Enschede, The Netherlands

*Address all correspondence to: n.a.van_de_zande@lumc.nl

References

[1] MacDonald ME, Ambrose CM, Duyao MP, Myers RH, Lin C, Srinidhi L, et al. A novel gene containing a trinucleotide repeat that is expanded and unstable on Huntington's disease chromosomes. Cell. 1993;**72**(6):971-983

[2] Unified Huntington's disease rating scale: Reliability and consistency. Movement Disorders. 1996;**11**(2):136-142

[3] Craufurd D, Snowden J. Neuropsychological and neuropsychiatric aspects of Huntington's disease. Oxford Monographs on Medical Genetics. 2002;**45**:62-94

[4] Tabrizi SJ, Reilmann R, Roos RAC, Durr A, Leavitt B, Owen G, et al. Potential endpoints for clinical trials in premanifest and early Huntington's disease in the TRACK-HD study: Analysis of 24 month observational data. The Lancet Neurology. 2012;**11**(1):42-53

[5] Atkinson AJCW, DeGruttola VG, Demets DL, Downing GJ, Hoth DF, et al. Biomarkers and surrogate endpoints: Preferred definitions and conceptual framework. Clinical Pharmacology and Therapeutics. 2001;**69**(3):89-95

[6] Penney JB Jr, Vonsattel J-P, Macdonald ME, Gusella JF, Myers RH. CAG repeat number governs the development rate of pathology in Huntington's disease. Annals of Neurology. 1997;**41**(5):689-692

[7] Sun Y-M, Zhang Y-B, Wu Z-Y. Huntington's disease: Relationship between phenotype and genotype. Molecular Neurobiology. 2017;**54**(1): 342-348

[8] Chao TK, Hu J, Pringsheim T. Risk factors for the onset and progression of Huntington disease. Neurotoxicology. 2017;**61**:79-99

[9] Davies SW, Turmaine M, Cozens BA, DiFiglia M, Sharp AH, Ross CA, et al. Formation of neuronal Intranuclear inclusions underlies the neurological dysfunction in mice transgenic for the HD mutation. Cell. 1997;**90**(3):537-548

[10] Li SH, Cheng AL, Zhou H, Lam S, Rao M, Li H, et al. Interaction of Huntington disease protein with transcriptional activator Sp1. Molecular and Cellular Biology. 2002;**22**(5):1277-1287

[11] Vonsattel J-P, Myers RH, Stevens TJ, Ferrante RJ, Bird ED, Richardson EP Jr. Neuropathological classification of Huntington's disease. Journal of Neuropathology & Experimental Neurology. 1985;**44**(6):559-577

[12] de la Monte SM, Vonsattel J-P, Richardson EP Jr. Morphometric demonstration of atrophic changes in the cerebral cortex, white matter, and neostriatum in Huntington's disease. Journal of Neuropathology & Experimental Neurology. 1988; **47**(5):516-525

[13] Reiner A, Albin RL, Anderson KD, D'Amato CJ, Penney JB, Young AB. Differential loss of striatal projection neurons in Huntington disease. Proceedings of the National Academy of Sciences of the United States of America. 1988;**85**(15):5733-5737

[14] Estrada-Sánchez AM, Rebec GV. Role of cerebral cortex in the neuropathology of Huntington's disease. Front Neural Circuits. 2013;7:19

[15] Rüb U, Vonsattel JP, Heinsen H, Korf HW. The

neuropathology of Huntington's disease: Classical findings, recent developments and correlation to functional neuroanatomy. Advances in Anatomy, Embryology, and Cell Biology. 2015;**217**:1-146

[16] Rüb U, Seidel K, Heinsen H, Vonsattel JP, den Dunnen WF, Korf HW. Huntington's disease (HD): The neuropathology of a multisystem neurodegenerative disorder of the human brain. Brain Pathology. 2016;**26**(6):726-740

[17] Rüb U, Hoche F, Brunt ER, Heinsen H, Seidel K, Del Turco D, et al. Degeneration of the cerebellum in Huntington's disease (HD): Possible relevance for the clinical picture and potential gateway to pathological mechanisms of the disease process. Brain Pathology. 2013;**23**(2):165-177

[18] Hu H, McCaw EA, Hebb ALO, Gomez GT, Denovan-Wright EM. Mutant huntingtin affects the rate of transcription of striatum-specific isoforms of phosphodiesterase 10A. European Journal of Neuroscience. 2004;**20**(12):3351-3363

[19] Hebb A, Robertson H, Denovan-Wright E. Striatal phosphodiesterase mRNA and protein levels are reduced in Huntington's disease transgenic mice prior to the onset of motor symptoms. Neuroscience. 2004;**123**:967-981

[20] Perry TL, Hansen S, Kloster M. Huntington's chorea. Deficiency of gamma-aminobutyric acid in brain. The New England Journal of Medicine. 1973;**288**(7):337-342

[21] Penney JB, Young AB. Quantitative autoradiography of neurotransmitter receptors in Huntington disease. Neurology. 1982;**32**(12):1391

[22] Lee CF, Chern Y. Adenosine receptors and Huntington's disease. International Review of Neurobiology. 2014;**119**:195-232

[23] Cristino L, Bisogno T, Di Marzo V. Cannabinoids and the expanded endocannabinoid system in neurological disorders. Nature Reviews. Neurology. 2020;**16**(1):9-29

[24] Laprairie RB, Bagher AM, Rourke JL, Zrein A, Cairns EA, Kelly MEM, et al. Positive allosteric modulation of the type 1 cannabinoid receptor reduces the signs and symptoms of Huntington's disease in the R6/2 mouse model. Neuropharmacology. 2019;**151**:1-12

[25] Kuhn A, Goldstein DR, Hodges A, Strand AD, Sengstag T, Kooperberg C, et al. Mutant huntingtin's effects on striatal gene expression in mice recapitulate changes observed in human Huntington's disease brain and do not differ with mutant huntingtin length or wild-type huntingtin dosage. Human Molecular Genetics. 2007;**16**(15):1845-1861

[26] Ooms M, Rietjens R, Rangarajan JR, Vunckx K, Valdeolivas S, Maes F, et al. Early decrease of type 1 cannabinoid receptor binding and phosphodiesterase 10A activity in vivo in R6/2 Huntington mice. Neurobiology of Aging. 2014;**35**(12):2858-2869

[27] Muller M, Leavitt BR. Iron dysregulation in Huntington's disease. Journal of Neurochemistry. 2014;**130**(3):328-350

[28] Deng YP, Wong T, Bricker-Anthony C, Deng B, Reiner A. Loss of corticostriatal and thalamostriatal synaptic terminals precedes striatal projection neuron pathology in heterozygous Q140 Huntington's disease mice. Neurobiology of Disease. 2013;**60**:89-107

[29] DiProspero NA, Chen EY, Charles V, Plomann M, Kordower JH, Tagle DA. Early changes in Huntington's disease patient brains involve alterations in cytoskeletal and synaptic elements. Journal of Neurocytology. 2004;**33**(5):517-533

[30] Carmo C, Naia L, Lopes C, Rego AC. Mitochondrial dysfunction in Huntington's disease. Advances in Experimental Medicine and Biology. 2018;**1049**:59-83

[31] Simmons DA, Casale M, Alcon B, Pham N, Narayan N, Lynch G. Ferritin accumulation in dystrophic microglia is an early event in the development of Huntington's disease. Glia. 2007;**55**(10):1074-1084

[32] Sapp E, Kegel KB, Aronin N, Hashikawa T, Uchiyama Y, Tohyama K, et al. Early and progressive accumulation of reactive microglia in the Huntington disease brain. Journal of Neuropathology and Experimental Neurology. 2001;**60**(2):161-172

[33] Currie S, Hoggard N, Craven IJ, Hadjivassiliou M, Wilkinson ID. Understanding MRI: Basic MR physics for physicians. Postgraduate Medical Journal. 2013;**89**(1050):209-223

[34] Johnson EB, Gregory S. Huntington's disease: Brain imaging in Huntington's disease. In: Brain Imaging. Progress in Molecular Biology and Translational Science. Elsevier; 2019. pp. 321-369. DOI: 10.1016/bs.pmbts.2019.04.004

[35] Ashburner J, Friston KJ. Voxel-based morphometry—The methods. NeuroImage. 2000;**11**(6):805-821

[36] Smith SM, Jenkinson M, Johansen-Berg H, Rueckert D, Nichols TE, Mackay CE, et al. Tract-based spatial statistics: Voxelwise analysis of multi-subject diffusion data. NeuroImage. 2006;**31**(4):1487-1505

[37] Heinen R, Bouvy WH, Mendrik AM, Viergever MA, Biessels GJ, de Bresser J. Robustness of automated methods for brain volume measurements across different MRI Field strengths. PLoS One. 2016;**11**(10):e0165719

[38] Harris GJ, Pearlson GD, Peyser CE, Aylward EH, Roberts J, Barta PE, et al. Putamen volume reduction on magnetic resonance imaging exceeds caudate changes in mild Huntington's disease. Annals of Neurology. 1992;**31**(1):69-75

[39] Harris GJ, Aylward EH, Peyser CE, Pearlson GD, Brandt J, Roberts-Twillie JV, et al. Single photon emission computed tomographic blood flow and magnetic resonance volume imaging of basal ganglia in Huntington's disease. Archives of Neurology. 1996;**53**(4):316-324

[40] Aylward EH, Codori A-M, Barta PE, Pearlson GD, Harris GJ, Brandt J. Basal ganglia volume and proximity to onset in presymptomatic Huntington disease. Archives of Neurology. 1996;**53**(12):1293-1296

[41] Aylward EH. Magnetic resonance imaging striatal volumes: A biomarker for clinical trials in Huntington's disease. Movement Disorders. 2014;**29**(11):1429-1433

[42] Aylward EH, Sparks BF, Field KM, Yallapragada V, Shpritz BD, Rosenblatt A, et al. Onset and rate of striatal atrophy in preclinical Huntington disease. Neurology. 2004;**63**(1):66-72

[43] Tabrizi SJ, Langbehn DR, Leavitt BR, Roos RAC, Durr A, Craufurd D, et al. Biological and clinical manifestations of Huntington's disease in the longitudinal TRACK-HD study: Cross-sectional analysis of baseline data. The Lancet Neurology. 2009;**8**(9):791-801

[44] Paulsen JS, Hayden M, Stout JC, Langbehn DR, Aylward E, Ross CA, et al. Preparing for preventive clinical trials: The predict-HD study. Archives of Neurology. 2006;**63**(6):883-890

[45] Bogaard SJA, Dumas EM, Acharya TP, Johnson H, Langbehn DR, Scahill RI, et al. Early atrophy of pallidum and accumbens nucleus in Huntington's disease. Journal of Neurology. 2010;**258**(3):412-420

[46] Aylward EH, Nopoulos PC, Ross CA, Langbehn DR, Pierson RK, Mills JA, et al. Longitudinal change in regional brain volumes in prodromal Huntington disease. Journal of Neurology, Neurosurgery & Psychiatry. 2011;**82**(4):405-410

[47] Paulsen JS, Langbehn DR, Stout JC, Aylward E, Ross CA, Nance M, et al. Detection of Huntington's disease decades before diagnosis: The predict-HD study. Journal of Neurology, Neurosurgery & Psychiatry. 2008;**79**(8):874-880

[48] Hobbs NZ, Barnes J, Frost C, Henley SMD, Wild EJ, Macdonald K, et al. Onset and progression of pathologic atrophy in Huntington disease: A longitudinal MR imaging study. American Journal of Neuroradiology. 2010;**31**(6):1036-1041

[49] Tabrizi SJ, Scahill RI, Durr A, Roos RAC, Leavitt BR, Jones R, et al. Biological and clinical changes in premanifest and early stage Huntington's disease in the TRACK-HD study: The 12-month longitudinal analysis. The Lancet Neurology. 2011;**10**(1):31-42

[50] Tabrizi SJ, Scahill RI, Owen G, Durr A, Leavitt BR, Roos RA, et al. Predictors of phenotypic progression and disease onset in premanifest and early-stage Huntington's disease in the TRACK-HD study: Analysis of 36-month observational data. The Lancet Neurology. 2013;**12**(7):637-649

[51] Draganski B, Domínguez DJF, Egan GF, Gray MA, Poudel GR, Churchyard A, et al. Multi-modal neuroimaging in premanifest and early Huntington's disease: 18 month longitudinal data from the IMAGE-HD study. PLoS One. 2013;**8**(9):e74131. DOI: 10.1371/journal.pone.0074131

[52] Aylward EH, Anderson NB, Bylsma FW, Wagster MV, Barta PE, Sherr M, et al. Frontal lobe volume in patients with Huntington's disease. Neurology. 1998;**50**(1):252-258

[53] Rosas HD, Koroshetz WJ, Chen YI, Skeuse C, Vangel M, Cudkowicz ME, et al. Evidence for more widespread cerebral pathology in early HD. An MRI-based morphometric analysis. Neurology. 2003;**60**(10):1615-1620

[54] Ciarmiello A, Cannella M, Lastoria S, Simonelli M, Frati L, Rubinsztein DC, et al. Brain white-matter volume loss and glucose hypometabolism precede the clinical symptoms of Huntington's disease. Journal of Nuclear Medicine. 2006;**47**(2):215-222

[55] Ruocco HH, Bonilha L, Li LM, Lopes-Cendes I, Cendes F. Longitudinal analysis of regional grey matter loss in Huntington disease: Effects of the length of the expanded CAG repeat. Journal of Neurology, Neurosurgery & Psychiatry. 2008;**79**(2):130-135

[56] Paulsen JS, Nopoulos PC, Aylward E, Ross CA, Johnson H, Magnotta VA, et al. Striatal and white matter predictors of estimated diagnosis for Huntington disease. Brain Research Bulletin. 2010;**82**(3-4):201-207

[57] Delva A, Michiels L, Koole M, Van Laere K, Vandenberghe W. Synaptic

damage and its clinical correlates in people with early Huntington disease: A PET study. Neurology. 2021;**98**(1):e83-e94

[58] Rosas HD, Liu AK, Hersch S, Glessner M, Ferrante RJ, Salat DH, et al. Regional and progressive thinning of the cortical ribbon in Huntington's disease. Neurology. 2002;**58**(5):695-701

[59] Rosas HD, Salat DH, Lee SY, Zaleta AK, Pappu V, Fischl B, et al. Cerebral cortex and the clinical expression of Huntington's disease: Complexity and heterogeneity. Brain. 2008;**131**(4):1057-1068

[60] Coppen EM, Grond JV, Hafkemeijer A, Barkey Wolf JJH, Roos RAC. Structural and functional changes of the visual cortex in early Huntington's disease. Human Brain Mapping. 2018;**39**(12):4776-4786

[61] Rosas HD, Goodman J, Chen YI, Jenkins BG, Kennedy DN, Makris N, et al. Striatal volume loss in HD as measured by MRI and the influence of CAG repeat. Neurology. 2001;**57**(6):1025-1028

[62] Ceccarini J, Ahmad R, Van de Vliet L, Casteels C, Vandenbulcke M, Vandenberghe W, et al. Behavioral symptoms in premanifest Huntington disease correlate with reduced frontal CB1R levels. Journal of Nuclear Medicine. 2019;**60**(1):115-121

[63] Frost C, Mulick A, Scahill RI, Owen G, Aylward E, Leavitt BR, et al. Design optimization for clinical trials in early-stage manifest Huntington's disease. Movement Disorders. 2017;**32**(11):1610-1619

[64] Hobbs NZ, Farmer RE, Rees EM, Cole JH, Haider S, Malone IB, et al. Short-interval observational data to inform clinical trial design in Huntington's disease. Journal of Neurology, Neurosurgery & Psychiatry. 2015;**86**(12):1291-1298

[65] Aylward EH, Harrington DL, Mills JA, Nopoulos PC, Ross CA, Long JD, et al. Regional atrophy associated with cognitive and motor function in prodromal Huntington disease. Journal of Huntington's Disease. 2013;**2**:477-489

[66] Bechtel N, Scahill RI, Rosas HD, Acharya T, van den Bogaard SJA, Jauffret C, et al. Tapping linked to function and structure in premanifest and symptomatic Huntington disease. Neurology. 2010;**75**(24):2150-2160

[67] Scahill RI, Hobbs NZ, Say MJ, Bechtel N, Henley SMD, Hyare H, et al. Clinical impairment in premanifest and early Huntington's disease is associated with regionally specific atrophy. Human Brain Mapping. 2013;**34**:519-529

[68] Rosas HD, Hevelone ND, Zaleta AK, Greve DN, Salat DH, Fischl B. Regional cortical thinning in preclinical Huntington disease and its relationship to cognition. Neurology. 2005;**65**(5):745-747

[69] Garcia-Gorro C, Llera A, Martinez-Horta S, Perez-Perez J, Kulisevsky J, Rodriguez-Dechicha N, et al. Specific patterns of brain alterations underlie distinct clinical profiles in Huntington's disease. NeuroImage: Clinical. 2019;**23**. DOI: 10.1016/j.nicl.2019.101900

[70] Sweidan W, Bao F, Bozorgzad NS, George E. White and Gray matter abnormalities in manifest Huntington's disease: Cross-sectional and longitudinal analysis. Journal of Neuroimaging. 2020;**30**(3):351-358

[71] Johnson EB, Rees EM, Labuschagne I, Durr A, Leavitt BR, Roos RA, et al. The

impact of occipital lobe cortical thickness on cognitive task performance: An investigation in Huntington's disease. Neuropsychologia. 2015;**79**(Pt A): 138-146

[72] Labuschagne I, Cassidy AM, Scahill RI, Johnson EB, Rees E, O'Regan A, et al. Visuospatial processing deficits linked to posterior brain regions in Premanifest and early stage Huntington's disease. Journal of the International Neuropsychological Society. 2016;**22**(6):595-608

[73] Sampedro F, Martínez-Horta S, Perez-Perez J, Horta-Barba A, Lopez-Mora DA, Camacho V, et al. Cortical atrophic-hypometabolic dissociation in the transition from premanifest to early-stage Huntington's disease. European Journal of Nuclear Medicine and Molecular Imaging. 2019;**46**(5):1111-1116

[74] Douaud G, Gaura V, Ribeiro MJ, Lethimonnier F, Maroy R, Verny C, et al. Distribution of grey matter atrophy in Huntington's disease patients: A combined ROI-based and voxel-based morphometric study. NeuroImage. 2006;**32**(4):1562-1575

[75] Jech R, Klempíř J, Vymazal J, Židovská J, Klempířová O, Růžička E, et al. Variation of selective gray and white matter atrophy in Huntington's disease. Movement Disorders. 2007;**22**(12):1783-1789

[76] Baake V, Coppen EM, van Duijn E, Dumas EM, van den Bogaard SJA, Scahill RI, et al. Apathy and atrophy of subcortical brain structures in Huntington's disease: A two-year follow-up study. NeuroImage: Clinical. 2018;**19**:66-70

[77] Peinemann A, Schuller S, Pohl C, Jahn T, Weindl A, Kassubek J. Executive dysfunction in early stages of Huntington's disease is associated with striatal and insular atrophy: A neuropsychological and voxel-based morphometric study. Journal of the Neurological Sciences. 2005;**239**(1):11-19

[78] Kassubek J, Juengling FD, Ecker D, Landwehrmeyer GB. Thalamic atrophy in Huntington's disease co-varies with cognitive performance: A morphometric MRI analysis. Cerebral Cortex. 2005;**15**(6):846-853

[79] Le Bihan D, Mangin J-F, Poupon C, Clark CA, Pappata S, Molko N, et al. Diffusion tensor imaging: Concepts and applications. Journal of Magnetic Resonance Imaging. 2001;**13**(4):534-546

[80] Gatto RG, Weissmann C. Diffusion tensor imaging in preclinical and human studies of Huntington's disease: What have we learned so far? Current Medical Imaging Formerly Current Medical Imaging Reviews. 2019;**15**(6):521-542

[81] van den Bogaard SJA, Dumas EM, van der Grond J, van Buchem MA, Roos RAC. MRI biomarkers in Huntington's disease. Frontiers in Bioscience. 2012;**4**:1910-1925

[82] Rosas HD, Wilkens P, Salat DH, Mercaldo ND, Vangel M, Yendiki AY, et al. Complex spatial and temporally defined myelin and axonal degeneration in Huntington disease. NeuroImage: Clinical. 2018;**20**:236-242

[83] Garcia-Gorro C, de Diego-Balaguer R, Martínez-Horta S, Pérez-Pérez J, Kulisevsky J, Rodríguez-Dechicha N, et al. Reduced striato-cortical and inhibitory transcallosal connectivity in the motor circuit of Huntington's disease patients. Human Brain Mapping. 2018;**39**(1):54-71

[84] Shaffer JJ, Ghayoor A, Long JD, Kim RE-Y, Lourens S, O'Donnell LJ, et al. Longitudinal diffusion changes in

prodromal and early HD: Evidence of white-matter tract deterioration. Human Brain Mapping. 2017;**38**(3):1460-1477

[85] Phillips OR, Joshi SH, Squitieri F, Sanchez-Castaneda C, Narr K, Shattuck DW, et al. Major superficial white matter abnormalities in Huntington's disease. Frontiers in Neuroscience. 2016;**10**(197). DOI: 10.3389/fnins.2016.00197

[86] Steventon JJ, Trueman RC, Rosser AE, Jones DK. Robust MR-based approaches to quantifying white matter structure and structure/function alterations in Huntington's disease. Journal of Neuroscience Methods. 2016;**265**:2-12

[87] Matsui JT, Vaidya JG, Wassermann D, Kim RE, Magnotta VA, Johnson HJ, et al. Prefrontal cortex white matter tracts in prodromal Huntington disease. Human Brain Mapping. 2015;**36**(10):3717-3732

[88] Odish OFF, Caeyenberghs K, Hosseini H, van den Bogaard SJA, Roos RAC, Leemans A. Dynamics of the connectome in Huntington's disease: A longitudinal diffusion MRI study. NeuroImage: Clinical. 2015;**9**:32-43

[89] Della Nave R, Ginestroni A, Tessa C, Giannelli M, Piacentini S, Filippi M, et al. Regional distribution and clinical correlates of white matter structural damage in Huntington disease: A tract-based spatial statistics study. American Journal of Neuroradiology. 2010;**31**(9):1675-1681

[90] Zhang J, Gregory S, Scahill RI, Durr A, Thomas DL, Lehericy S, et al. In vivo characterization of white matter pathology in premanifest Huntington's disease. Annals of Neurology. 2018;**84**(4):497-504

[91] Bohanna I, Georgiou-Karistianis N, Sritharan A, Asadi H, Johnston L, Churchyard A, et al. Diffusion tensor imaging in Huntington's disease reveals distinct patterns of white matter degeneration associated with motor and cognitive deficits. Brain Imaging and Behavior. 2011;**5**(3):171-180

[92] Reading SAJ, Yassa MA, Bakker A, Dziorny AC, Gourley LM, Yallapragada V, et al. Regional white matter change in pre-symptomatic Huntington's disease: A diffusion tensor imaging study. Psychiatry Research: Neuroimaging. 2005;**140**(1):55-62

[93] McColgan P, Seunarine KK, Gregory S, Razi A, Papoutsi M, Long JD, et al. Topological length of white matter connections predicts their rate of atrophy in premanifest Huntington's disease. JCI Insight. 2017;**2**(8):e92641. DOI: 10.1172/jci.insight.92641

[94] Rosas HD, Lee SY, Bender AC, Zaleta AK, Vangel M, Yu P, et al. Altered white matter microstructure in the corpus callosum in Huntington's disease: Implications for cortical "disconnection". NeuroImage. 2010;**49**(4):2995-3004

[95] Wu D, Faria AV, Younes L, Mori S, Brown T, Johnson H, et al. Mapping the order and pattern of brain structural MRI changes using change-point analysis in premanifest Huntington's disease. Human Brain Mapping. 2017;**38**(10):5035-5050

[96] Liu W, Yang J, Burgunder J, Cheng B, Shang H. Diffusion imaging studies of Huntington's disease: A meta-analysis. Parkinsonism & Related Disorders. 2016;**32**:94-101

[97] Müller H-P, Gorges M, Grön G, Kassubek J, Landwehrmeyer GB, Süßmuth SD, et al. Motor network structure and function are associated with motor performance in Huntington's

disease. Journal of Neurology. 2016;**263**(3):539-549

[98] Müller HP, Grön G, Sprengelmeyer R, Kassubek J, Ludolph AC, Hobbs N, et al. Evaluating multicenter DTI data in Huntington's disease on site specific effects: An ex post facto approach. Neuroimage Clinical. 2013;**2**:161-167

[99] Müller H-P, Kassubek J, Grön G, Sprengelmeyer R, Ludolph A, Klöppel S, et al. Diffusion tensor imaging In Huntington's disease: Impact of the control for corrupted data in comparisons at the group level. Biomedical Engineering Online. 2014;**13**:128

[100] Delmaire C, Dumas EM, Sharman MA, van den Bogaard SJA, Valabregue R, Jauffret C, et al. The structural correlates of functional deficits in early huntington's disease. Human Brain Mapping. 2013;**34**(9):2141-2153

[101] Hobbs NZ, Cole JH, Farmer RE, Rees EM, Crawford HE, Malone IB, et al. Evaluation of multi-modal, multi-site neuroimaging measures in Huntington's disease: Baseline results from the PADDINGTON study. NeuroImage Clinical [Internet]. 2012;**2**:204-211

[102] Klöppel S, Draganski B, Golding CV, Chu C, Nagy Z, Cook PA, et al. White matter connections reflect changes in voluntary-guided saccades in pre-symptomatic Huntington's disease. Brain. 2008;**131**(1):196-204

[103] Rosas HD, Tuch DS, Hevelone ND, Zaleta AK, Vangel M, Hersch SM, et al. Diffusion tensor imaging in presymptomatic and early Huntington's disease: Selective white matter pathology and its relationship to clinical measures. Movement Disorders. 2006;**21**(9):1317-1325

[104] Pflanz CP, Charquero-Ballester M, Majid DSA, Winkler AM, Vallée E, Aron AR, et al. One-year changes in brain microstructure differentiate preclinical Huntington's disease stages. NeuroImage: Clinical. 2020;**25**. DOI: 10.1016/j.nicl.2019.102099

[105] Pini L, Youssov K, Sambataro F, Bachoud-Levi AC, Vallesi A, Jacquemot C. Striatal connectivity in pre-manifest Huntington's disease is differentially affected by disease burden. European Journal of Neurology. 2020;**27**(11):2147-2157

[106] Syka M, Keller J, Klempíř J, Rulseh AM, Roth J, Jech R, et al. Correlation between relaxometry and diffusion tensor imaging in the globus pallidus of Huntington's disease patients. PLoS One. 2015;**10**(3):e0118907-e

[107] Poudel GR, Stout JC, Domínguez DJF, Churchyard A, Chua P, Egan GF, et al. Longitudinal change in white matter microstructure in Huntington's disease: The IMAGE-HD study. Neurobiology of Disease. 2015;**74**:406-412

[108] Matsui JT, Vaidya JG, Johnson HJ, Magnotta VA, Long JD, Mills JA, et al. Diffusion weighted imaging of prefrontal cortex in prodromal Huntington's disease. Human Brain Mapping. 2014;**35**(4):1562-1573

[109] Domínguez DJF, Stout JC, Poudel G, Churchyard A, Chua P, Egan GF, et al. Multimodal imaging biomarkers in premanifest and early Huntington's disease: 30-month IMAGE-HD data. The British Journal of Psychiatry. 2016;**208**(6):571-578

[110] Sampedro F, Martínez-Horta S, Perez-Perez J, Horta-Barba A, Martin-Lahoz J, Alonso-Solís A, et al. Widespread increased diffusivity

reveals early cortical degeneration in Huntington disease. American Journal of Neuroradiology. 2019;**40**(9):1464-1468

[111] Domínguez DJF, Egan GF, Gray MA, Poudel GR, Churchyard A, Chua P, et al. Multi-modal neuroimaging in premanifest and early Huntington's disease: 18 month longitudinal data from the IMAGE-HD study. PLoS One. 2013;**8**(9):e74131

[112] Sritharan A, Egan GF, Johnston L, Horne M, Bradshaw JL, Bohanna I, et al. A longitudinal diffusion tensor imaging study in symptomatic Huntington's disease. Journal of Neurology, Neurosurgery & Psychiatry. 2009;**81**(3):257-262

[113] Vandenberghe W, Demaerel P, Dom R, Maes F. Diffusion-weighted versus volumetric imaging of the striatum in early symptomatic Huntington disease. Journal of Neurology. 2009;**256**(1):109-114

[114] Poudel GR, Stout JC, Domínguez DJF, Salmon L, Churchyard A, Chua P, et al. White matter connectivity reflects clinical and cognitive status in Huntington's disease. Neurobiology of Disease. 2014;**65**:180-187

[115] Phillips O, Sanchez-Castaneda C, Elifani F, Maglione V, Di Pardo A, Caltagirone C, et al. Tractography of the corpus callosum in Huntington's disease. PLoS One. 2013;**8**(9):e73280

[116] De Paepe AE, Sierpowska J, Garcia-Gorro C, Martinez-Horta S, Perez-Perez J, Kulisevsky J, et al. White matter cortico-striatal tracts predict apathy subtypes in Huntington's disease. NeuroImage: Clinical. 2019;**24**:101965. DOI: 10.1016/j.nicl.2019.101965

[117] Gregory S, Scahill RI, Seunarine KK, Stopford C, Zhang H, Zhang J, et al. Neuropsychiatry and white matter microstructure in Huntington's disease. Journal of Huntington's Disease. 2015;**4**(3):239-249

[118] Georgiou-Karistianis N, Gray MA, Domínguez DJF, Dymowski AR, Bohanna I, Johnston LA, et al. Automated differentiation of pre-diagnosis Huntington's disease from healthy control individuals based on quadratic discriminant analysis of the basal ganglia: The IMAGE-HD study. Neurobiology of Disease. 2013;**51**:82-92

[119] Gujar SK, Maheshwari S, Björkman-Burtscher I, Sundgren PC. Magnetic resonance spectroscopy. Journal of Neuro-Ophthalmology. 2005;**25**(3):217-226

[120] Reynolds NC Jr, Prost RW, Mark LP. Heterogeneity in 1H-MRS profiles of presymptomatic and early manifest Huntington's disease. Brain Research. 2005;**1031**(1):82-89

[121] Sturrock A, Laule C, Decolongon J, Dar Santos R, Coleman AJ, Creighton S, et al. Magnetic resonance spectroscopy biomarkers in premanifest and early Huntington disease. Neurology. 2010;**75**(19):1702-1710

[122] Clarke CE, Lowry M, Quarrell OW. No change in striatal glutamate in Huntington's disease measured by proton magnetic resonance spectroscopy. Parkinsonism & Related Disorders. 1998;**4**(3):123-127

[123] Jenkins BG, Koroshetz WJ, Beal MF, Rosen BR. Evidence for impairment of energy metabolism in vivo in Huntington's disease using localized 1H NMR spectroscopy. Neurology. 1993;**43**(12):2689-2695

[124] Jenkins BG, Rosas HD, Chen YC, Makabe T, Myers R, MacDonald M,

et al. 1H NMR spectroscopy studies of Huntington's disease: Correlations with CAG repeat numbers. Neurology. 1998;**50**(5):1357-1365

[125] Sánchez-Pernaute R, García-Segura JM, del Barrio AA, Viaño J, de Yébenes JG. Clinical correlation of striatal 1H MRS changes in Huntington's disease. Neurology. 1999;**53**(4):806-812

[126] Ruocco HH, Lopes-Cendes I, Li LM, Cendes F. Evidence of thalamic dysfunction in Huntington disease by proton magnetic resonance spectroscopy. Movement Disorders. 2007;**22**(14):2052-2056

[127] Adanyeguh IM, Monin ML, Rinaldi D, Freeman L, Durr A, Lehéricy S, et al. Expanded neurochemical profile in the early stage of Huntington disease using proton magnetic resonance spectroscopy. NMR in Biomedicine. 2018;**31**(3). DOI: 10.1002/nbm.3880

[128] Gómez-Ansón B, Alegret M, Muñoz E, Sainz A, Monte GC, Tolosa E. Decreased frontal choline and neuropsychological performance in preclinical Huntington disease. Neurology. 2007;**68**(12):906-910

[129] van Oostrom JC, Sijens PE, Roos RA, Leenders KL. 1H magnetic resonance spectroscopy in preclinical Huntington disease. Brain Research. 2007;**1168**:67-71

[130] Taylor-Robinson SD, Weeks RA, Bryant DJ, Sargentoni J, Marcus CD, Harding AE, et al. Proton magnetic resonance spectroscopy in Huntington's disease: Evidence in favour of the glutamate excitotoxic theory. Movement Disorders. 1996;**11**(2):167-173

[131] Taylor-Robinson SD, Weeks RA, Sargentoni J, Marcus CD, Bryant DJ, Harding AE, et al. Evidence for glutamate excitotoxicity in Huntington's disease with proton magnetic resonance spectroscopy. Lancet. 1994;**343**(8906):1170

[132] Davie CA, Barker GJ, Quinn N, Tofts PS, Miller DH. Proton MRS in Huntington's disease. Lancet. 1994;**343**(8912):1580

[133] Harms L, Meierkord H, Timm G, Pfeiffer L, Ludolph AC. Decreased N-acetyl-aspartate/choline ratio and increased lactate in the frontal lobe of patients with Huntington's disease: A proton magnetic resonance spectroscopy study. Journal of Neurology, Neurosurgery, and Psychiatry. 1997;**62**(1):27-30

[134] Martin WR, Wieler M, Hanstock CC. Is brain lactate increased in Huntington's disease? Journal of the Neurological Sciences. 2007;**263**(1-2):70-74

[135] Sturrock A, Laule C, Wyper K, Milner RA, Decolongon J, Dar Santos R, et al. A longitudinal study of magnetic resonance spectroscopy Huntington's disease biomarkers. Movement Disorders. 2015;**30**(3):393-401

[136] Lowe AJ, Rodrigues FB, Arridge M, Johnson EB, Scahill RI, Byrne LM, et al. Longitudinal evaluation of magnetic resonance spectroscopy metabolites as biomarkers in Huntington's disease. medRxiv. 2021. DOI: 10.1101/2021.10.26.21265516

[137] Bartzokis G, Cummings J, Perlman S, Hance DB, Mintz J. Increased basal ganglia iron levels in Huntington disease. Archives of Neurology. 1999;**56**(5):569-574

[138] Dumas EM, Versluis MJ, van den Bogaard SJ, van Osch MJ, Hart EP, van Roon-Mom WM, et al. Elevated brain

iron is independent from atrophy in Huntington's disease. NeuroImage. 2012;**61**(3):558-564

[139] Rosas HD, Chen YI, Doros G, Salat DH, Chen NK, Kwong KK, et al. Alterations in brain transition metals in Huntington disease: An evolving and intricate story. Archives of Neurology. 2012;**69**(7):887-893

[140] Vymazal J, Klempíř J, Jech R, Židovská J, Syka M, Růžička E, et al. MR relaxometry in Huntington's disease: Correlation between imaging, genetic and clinical parameters. Journal of the Neurological Sciences. 2007;**263**(1): 20-25

[141] Sánchez-Castañeda C, Cherubini A, Elifani F, Péran P, Orobello S, Capelli G, et al. Seeking Huntington disease biomarkers by multimodal, cross-sectional basal ganglia imaging. Human Brain Mapping. 2013;**34**(7):1625-1635

[142] Domínguez JF, Ng AC, Poudel G, Stout JC, Churchyard A, Chua P, et al. Iron accumulation in the basal ganglia in Huntington's disease: Cross-sectional data from the IMAGE-HD study. Journal of Neurology, Neurosurgery, and Psychiatry. 2016;**87**(5):545-549

[143] Chen L, Hua J, Ross CA, Cai S, van Zijl PCM, Li X. Altered brain iron content and deposition rate in Huntington's disease as indicated by quantitative susceptibility MRI. Journal of Neuroscience Research. 2018;**97**(4):467-479

[144] Sánchez-Castañeda C, Squitieri F, Di Paola M, Dayan M, Petrollini M, Sabatini U. The role of iron in gray matter degeneration in Huntington's disease: A magnetic resonance imaging study. Human Brain Mapping. 2015;**36**(1):50-66

[145] Apple AC, Possin KL, Satris G, Johnson E, Lupo JM, Jakary A, et al. Quantitative 7T phase imaging in premanifest Huntington disease. AJNR. American Journal of Neuroradiology. 2014;**35**(9):1707-1713

[146] Johnson EB, Parker CS, Scahill RI, Gregory S, Papoutsi M, Zeun P, et al. Altered iron and myelin in premanifest Huntington's disease more than 20 years before clinical onset: Evidence from the cross-sectional HD Young adult study. eBioMedicine. 2021;**65**:103266. DOI: 10.1016/j.ebiom.2021.103266

[147] van Bergen JM, Hua J, Unschuld PG, Lim IA, Jones CK, Margolis RL, et al. Quantitative susceptibility mapping suggests altered brain iron in premanifest Huntington disease. AJNR. American Journal of Neuroradiology. 2016;**37**(5):789-796

[148] Glover GH. Overview of functional magnetic resonance imaging. Neurosurgery Clinics of North America. 2011;**22**(2):133-vii

[149] Gregory S, Scahill RI. Functional magnetic resonance imaging in Huntington's disease. Imaging in movement disorders: Imaging in atypical parkinsonism and familial movement disorders. International Review of Neurobiology. 2018;**142**:381-408

[150] Quarantelli M, Salvatore E, Giorgio SMDA, Filla A, Cervo A, Russo CV, et al. Default-mode network changes in Huntington's disease: An integrated MRI study of functional connectivity and morphometry. PLoS One. 2013;**8**(8):e72159

[151] Dumas EM, van den Bogaard SJA, Hart EP, Soeter RP, van Buchem MA, van der Grond J, et al. Reduced functional brain connectivity prior to and after

disease onset in Huntington's disease. NeuroImage: Clinical. 2013;**2**:377-384

[152] Koenig KA, Lowe MJ, Harrington DL, Lin J, Durgerian S, Mourany L, et al. Functional connectivity of primary motor cortex is dependent on genetic burden in prodromal Huntington disease. Brain Connectivity. 2014;**4**(7):535-546

[153] Unschuld PG, Joel SE, Pekar JJ, Reading SA, Oishi K, McEntee J, et al. Depressive symptoms in prodromal Huntington's disease correlate with Stroop-interference related functional connectivity in the ventromedial prefrontal cortex. Psychiatry Research: Neuroimaging. 2012;**203**(2):166-174

[154] Poudel GR, Egan GF, Churchyard A, Chua P, Stout JC, Georgiou-Karistianis N. Abnormal synchrony of resting state networks in premanifest and symptomatic Huntington disease: The IMAGE-HD study. Journal of Psychiatry and Neuroscience. 2014;**39**(2):87-96

[155] Wolf RC, Thomann PA, Sambataro F, Wolf ND, Vasic N, Landwehrmeyer GB, et al. Abnormal cerebellar volume and corticocerebellar dysfunction in early manifest Huntington's disease. Journal of Neurology. 2015;**262**(4):859-869

[156] Wolf RC, Sambataro F, Vasic N, Depping MS, Thomann PA, Landwehrmeyer GB, et al. Abnormal resting-state connectivity of motor and cognitive networks in early manifest Huntington's disease. Psychological Medicine. 2014;**44**(15):3341-3356

[157] Werner CJ, Dogan I, Saß C, Mirzazade S, Schiefer J, Shah NJ, et al. Altered resting-state connectivity in Huntington's disease. Human Brain Mapping. 2014;**35**(6):2582-2593

[158] Pini L, Jacquemot C, Cagnin A, Meneghello F, Semenza C, Mantini D, et al. Aberrant brain network connectivity in presymptomatic and manifest Huntington's disease: A systematic review. Human Brain Mapping. 2020;**41**(1):256-269

[159] McColgan P, Razi A, Gregory S, Seunarine KK, Durr A, Roos RAC, et al. Structural and functional brain network correlates of depressive symptoms in premanifest Huntington's disease. Human Brain Mapping. 2017;**38**(6):2819-2829

[160] Wolf RC, Sambataro F, Vasic N, WolfND,ThomannPA,LandwehrmeyerGB, et al. Longitudinal task-negative network analyses in preclinical Huntington's disease. European Archives of Psychiatry and Clinical Neuroscience. 2014;**264**(6):493-505

[161] Espinoza FA, Liu J, Ciarochi J, Turner JA, Vergara VM, Caprihan A, et al. Dynamic functional network connectivity in Huntington's disease and its associations with motor and cognitive measures. Human Brain Mapping. 2019;**40**(6):1955-1968

[162] Kronenbuerger M, Hua J, Bang Jee YA, Ultz K, Miao X, Zhang X, et al. Differential changes in functional connectivity of striatum-prefrontal and striatum-motor circuits in premanifest Huntington's disease. Neurodegenerative Diseases. 2019;**19**:1-10

[163] Gregory S, Long JD, Klöppel S, Razi A, Scheller E, Minkova L, et al. Testing a longitudinal compensation model in premanifest Huntington's disease. Brain. 2018;**141**(7):2156-2166

[164] Klöppel S, Gregory S, Scheller E, Minkova L, Razi A, Durr A, et al. Compensation in preclinical Huntington's disease: Evidence from the track-on HD study. eBioMedicine. 2015;**2**(10):1420-1429

[165] Odish OFF, van den Berg-Huysmans AA, van den Bogaard SJA, Dumas EM, Hart EP, Rombouts SARB, et al. Longitudinal resting state fMRI analysis in healthy controls and premanifest Huntington's disease gene carriers: A three-year follow-up study. Human Brain Mapping. 2015;**36**(1):110-119

[166] Seibert TM, Majid DSA, Aron AR, Corey-Bloom J, Brewer JB. Stability of resting fMRI interregional correlations analyzed in subject-native space: A one-year longitudinal study in healthy adults and premanifest Huntington's disease. NeuroImage. 2012;**59**(3):2452-2463

[167] Gargouri F, Messé A, Perlbarg V, Valabregue R, McColgan P, Yahia-Cherif L, et al. Longitudinal changes in functional connectivity of cortico-basal ganglia networks in manifests and premanifest huntington's disease. Human Brain Mapping. 2016;**37**(11):4112-4128

[168] Domínguez DJF, Poudel G, Stout JC, Gray M, Chua P, Borowsky B, et al. Longitudinal changes in the fronto-striatal network are associated with executive dysfunction and behavioral dysregulation in Huntington's disease: 30 months IMAGE-HD data. Cortex. 2017;**92**:139-149

[169] Georgiou-Karistianis N, Sritharan A, Farrow M, Cunnington R, Stout J, Bradshaw J, et al. Increased cortical recruitment in Huntington's disease using a Simon task. Neuropsychologia. 2007;**45**(8):1791-1800

[170] Georgiou-Karistianis N, Stout JC, Domínguez DJF, Carron SP, Ando A, Churchyard A, et al. Functional magnetic resonance imaging of working memory in Huntington's disease: Cross-sectional data from the IMAGE-HD study. Human Brain Mapping. 2014; **35**(5):1847-1864

[171] Wolf RC, Vasic N, Schönfeldt-Lecuona C, Ecker D, Landwehrmeyer GB. Cortical dysfunction in patients with Huntington's disease during working memory performance. Human Brain Mapping. 2009;**30**(1):327-339

[172] Klöppel S, Draganski B, Siebner HR, Tabrizi SJ, Weiller C, Frackowiak RSJ. Functional compensation of motor function in pre-symptomatic Huntington's disease. Brain. 2009;**132**(6):1624-1632

[173] Zimbelman JL, Paulsen JS, Mikos A, Reynolds NC, Hoffmann RG, Rao SM. fMRI detection of early neural dysfunction in preclinical Huntington's disease. Journal of the International Neuropsychological Society. 2007;**13**(5):758-769

[174] Paulsen JS, Zimbelman JL, Hinton SC, Langbehn DR, Leveroni CL, Benjamin ML, et al. fMRI biomarker of early neuronal dysfunction in presymptomatic Huntington's disease. American Journal of Neuroradiology. 2004;**25**(10):1715-1721

[175] Saft C, Lissek S, Hoffmann R, Nicolas V, Tegenthoff M, Juckel G, et al. Mentalizing in preclinical Huntington's disease: An fMRI study using cartoon picture stories. Brain Imaging and Behavior. 2013;**7**(2):154-162

[176] Wolf RC, Vasic N, Schönfeldt-Lecuona C, Landwehrmeyer GB, Ecker D. Dorsolateral prefrontal cortex dysfunction in presymptomatic Huntington's disease: Evidence from event-related fMRI. Brain. 2007;**130**(11):2845-2857

[177] Paulsen JS. Functional imaging in Huntington's disease. Experimental Neurology. 2009;**216**(2):272-277

[178] Poudel GR, Stout JC, Domínguez DJF, Gray MA, Salmon L,

Churchyard A, et al. Functional changes during working memory in Huntington's disease: 30-month longitudinal data from the IMAGE-HD study. Brain Structure and Function. 2015; **220**(1):501-512

[179] Georgiou-Karistianis N, Poudel GR, Domínguez DJF, Langmaid R, Gray MA, Churchyard A, et al. Functional and connectivity changes during working memory in Huntington's disease: 18month longitudinal data from the IMAGE-HD study. Brain and Cognition. 2013;**83**(1):80-91

[180] Wolf RC, Sambataro F, Vasic N, WolfND,ThomannPA,LandwehrmeyerGB, et al. Longitudinal functional magnetic resonance imaging of cognition in preclinical Huntington's disease. Experimental Neurology. 2011;**231**(2):214-222

[181] Gray MA, Egan GF, Ando A, Churchyard A, Chua P, Stout JC, et al. Prefrontal activity in Huntington's disease reflects cognitive and neuropsychiatric disturbances: The IMAGE-HD study. Experimental Neurology. 2013;**239**:218-228

[182] Cybulska K, Perk L, Booij J, Laverman P, Rijpkema M. Huntington's disease: A review of the known PET imaging biomarkers and targeting radiotracers. Molecules. 2020;**25**(3):482. DOI: 10.3390/molecules25030482

[183] Kuwert T, Lange HW, Langen K-J, Herzog H, Aulich A, Feinendegen LE. Cortical and subcortical glucose consumption measured by PET in patients with Huntington's disease. Brain. 1990;**113**(5):1405-1423

[184] Kuhl DE, Phelps ME, Markham CH, Metter EJ, Riege WH, Winter J. Cerebral metabolism and atrophy in huntington's disease determined by 18FDG and computed tomographic scan. Annals of Neurology. 1982;**12**(5):425-434

[185] Antonini A, Leenders KL, Spiegel R, Meier D, Vontobel P, Weigell-Weber M, et al. Striatal glucose metabolism and dopamine D2 receptor binding in asymptomatic gene carriers and patients with Huntington's disease. Brain. 1996;**119**(6):2085-2095

[186] Young AB, Penney JB, Starosta-Rubinstein S, Markel DS, Berent S, Giordani B, et al. PET scan investigations of Huntington's disease: Cerebral metabolic correlates of neurological features and functional decline. Annals of Neurology. 1986;**20**(3):296-303

[187] Feigin A, Leenders KL, Moeller JR, Missimer J, Kuenig G, Spetsieris P, et al. Metabolic network abnormalities in early Huntington's disease: An [(18)F]FDG PET study. Journal of Nuclear Medicine. 2001;**42**(11):1591-1595

[188] López-Mora DA, Camacho V, Pérez-Pérez J, Martínez-Horta S, Fernández A, Sampedro F, et al. Striatal hypometabolism in premanifest and manifest Huntington's disease patients. European Journal of Nuclear Medicine and Molecular Imaging. 2016;**43**(12):2183-2189

[189] Ciarmiello A, Giovacchini G, Orobello S, Bruselli L, Elifani F, Squitieri F. 18F-FDG PET uptake in the pre-Huntington disease caudate affects the time-to-onset independently of CAG expansion size. European Journal of Nuclear Medicine and Molecular Imaging. 2012;**39**(6):1030-1036

[190] Herben-Dekker M, van Oostrom JCH, Roos RAC, Jurgens CK, Witjes-Ané M-NW, Kremer HPH, et al. Striatal metabolism and psychomotor speed as predictors of motor onset

in Huntington's disease. Journal of Neurology. 2014;**261**(7):1387-1397

[191] Fernandez-Funez P, Hellem MNN, Vinther-Jensen T, Anderberg L, Budtz-Jørgensen E, Hjermind LE, et al. Hybrid 2-[18F] FDG PET/MRI in premanifest Huntington's disease gene-expansion carriers: The significance of partial volume correction. PLoS One. 2021;**16**(6). DOI: 10.1371/journal.pone.0252683

[192] Berent S, Giordani B, Lehtinen S, Markel D, Penney JB, Buchtel HA, et al. Positron emission tomographic scan investigations of Huntington's disease: Cerebral metabolic correlates of cognitive function. Annals of Neurology. 1988;**23**(6):541-546

[193] Tsuchida T, Sadato N, Nishizawa S, Yonekura Y, Itoh H. Effect of postprandial hyperglycaemia in non-invasive measurement of cerebral metabolic rate of glucose in non-diabetic subjects. European Journal of Nuclear Medicine and Molecular Imaging. 2002;**29**(2):248-250

[194] Foster NL, VanDerSpek AFL, Aldrich MS, Berent S, Hichwa RH, Sackellares JC, et al. The effect of diazepam sedation on cerebral glucose metabolism in Alzheimer's disease as measured using positron emission tomography. Journal of Cerebral Blood Flow & Metabolism. 1987;**7**(4):415-420

[195] Andrews TC, Weeks RA, Turjanski N, Gunn RN, Watkins LHA, Sahakian B, et al. Huntington's disease progression: PET and clinical observations. Brain. 1999;**122**(12):2353-2363

[196] Sedvall G, Karlsson P, Lundin A, Anvret M, Suhara T, Halldin C, et al. Dopamine D1 receptor number—A sensitive PET marker for early brain degeneration in Huntington's disease. European Archives of Psychiatry and Clinical Neuroscience. 1994;**243**(5):249-255

[197] Weeks RA, Piccini P, Harding AE, Brooks DJ. Striatal D1 and D2 dopamine receptor loss in asymptomatic mutation carriers of Huntington's disease. Annals of Neurology. 1996;**40**(1):49-54

[198] Turjanski N, Weeks R, Dolan R, Harding AE, Brooks DJ. Striatal D1 and D2 receptor binding in patients with Huntington's disease and other choreas: A PET study. Brain. 1995;**118**(3):689-696

[199] Ginovart N, Lundin A, Farde L, Halldin C, Bäckman L, Swahn CG, et al. PET study of the pre- and post-synaptic dopaminergic markers for the neurodegenerative process in Huntington's disease. Brain. 1997;**120**(3):503-514

[200] Pavese N, Andrews TC, Brooks DJ, Ho AK, Rosser AE, Barker RA, et al. Progressive striatal and cortical dopamine receptor dysfunction in Huntington's disease: A PET study. Brain. 2003;**126**(5):1127-1135

[201] van Oostrom JCH, Maguire RP, Verschuuren-Bemelmans CC, Veenma-van der Duin L, Pruim J, Roos RAC, et al. Striatal dopamine D2 receptors, metabolism, and volume in preclinical Huntington disease. Neurology. 2005;**65**(6):941-943

[202] Antonini A, Leenders KL, Eidelberg D. [11C]Raclopride-PET studies of the Huntington's disease rate of progression: Relevance of the trinucleotide repeat length. Annals of Neurology. 1998;**43**(2):253-255

[203] Lawrence AD, Weeks RA, Brooks DJ, Andrews TC, Watkins LH,

Harding AE, et al. The relationship between striatal dopamine receptor binding and cognitive performance in Huntington's disease. Brain. 1998;**121** (Pt 7):1343-1355

[204] Esmaeilzadeh M, Ciarmiello A, Squitieri F. Seeking brain biomarkers for preventive therapy in Huntington disease. CNS Neuroscience & Therapeutics. 2011;**17**(5):368-386

[205] Pavese N, Politis M, Tai YF, Barker RA, Tabrizi SJ, Mason SL, et al. Cortical dopamine dysfunction in symptomatic and premanifest Huntington's disease gene carriers. Neurobiology of Disease. 2010;**37**(2):356-361

[206] Politis M, Pavese N, Tai YF, Tabrizi SJ, Barker RA, Piccini P. Hypothalamic involvement in Huntington's disease: An in vivo PET study. Brain. 2008;**131**(11):2860-2869

[207] Niccolini F, Haider S, Reis Marques T, Muhlert N, Tziortzi AC, Searle GE, et al. Altered PDE10A expression detectable early before symptomatic onset in Huntington's disease. Brain. 2015;**138**(10):3016-3029

[208] Ahmad R, Bourgeois S, Postnov A, Schmidt ME, Bormans G, Van Laere K, et al. PET imaging shows loss of striatal PDE10A in patients with Huntington disease. Neurology. 2014;**82**(3):279-281

[209] Russell DS, Barret O, Jennings DL, Friedman JH, Tamagnan GD, Thomae D, et al. The phosphodiesterase 10 positron emission tomography tracer, [18F] MNI-659, as a novel biomarker for early Huntington disease. JAMA Neurology. 2014;**71**(12):1520-1528

[210] Russell DS, Jennings DL, Barret O, Tamagnan GD, Carroll VM, Caillé F, et al. Change in PDE10 across early Huntington disease assessed by [^{18}F]MNI-659 and PET imaging. Neurology. 2016;**86**(8):748-754

[211] Fazio P, Fitzer-Attas CJ, Mrzljak L, Bronzova J, Nag S, Warner JH, et al. PET molecular imaging of phosphodiesterase 10A: An early biomarker of Huntington's disease progression. Movement Disorders. 2020;**35**(4):606-615

[212] Van Laere K, Casteels C, Dhollander I, Goffin K, Grachev I, Bormans G, et al. Widespread decrease of type 1 cannabinoid receptor availability in Huntington disease in vivo. Journal of Nuclear Medicine. 2010;**51**(9):1413-1417

[213] Holthoff VA, Koeppe RA, Frey KA, Penney JB, Markel DS, Kuhl DE, et al. Positron emission tomography measures of benzodiazepine receptors in Huntington's disease. Annals of Neurology. 1993;**34**(1):76-81

[214] Künig G, Leenders KL, Sanchez-Pernaute R, Antonini A, Vontobel P, Verhagen A, et al. Benzodiazepine receptor binding in Huntington's disease: [11C]flumazenil uptake measured using positron emission tomography. Annals of Neurology. 2000;**47**(5):644-648

[215] Matusch A, Saft C, Elmenhorst D, Kraus PH, Gold R, Hartung H-P, et al. Cross sectional PET study of cerebral adenosine A1 receptors in premanifest and manifest Huntington's disease. European Journal of Nuclear Medicine and Molecular Imaging. 2014;**41**(6):1210-1220

[216] Pavese N, Gerhard A, Tai YF, Ho AK, Turkheimer F, Barker RA, et al. Microglial activation correlates with severity in Huntington disease. A clinical and PET study. Neurology. 2006;**66**(11):1638-1643

[217] Tai YF, Pavese N, Gerhard A, Tabrizi SJ, Barker RA, Brooks DJ, et al. Microglial activation in presymptomatic Huntington's disease gene carriers. Brain. 2007;**130**(7):1759-1766

[218] Lois C, González I, Izquierdo-García D, Zürcher NR, Wilkens P, Loggia ML, et al. Neuroinflammation in Huntington's disease: New insights with 11C-PBR28 PET/MRI. ACS Chemical Neuroscience. 2018;**9**(11):2563-2571

[219] Politis M, Pavese N, Tai YF, Kiferle L, Mason SL, Brooks DJ, et al. Microglial activation in regions related to cognitive function predicts disease onset in Huntington's disease: A multimodal imaging study. Human Brain Mapping. 2011;**32**(2):258-270

[220] Politis M, Lahiri N, Niccolini F, Su P, Wu K, Giannetti P, et al. Increased central microglial activation associated with peripheral cytokine levels in premanifest Huntington's disease gene carriers. Neurobiology of Disease. 2015;**83**:115-121

[221] CHDI Foundation I, Universitaire Ziekenhuizen L. iMagemHTT: FIH Evaluation of Novel Mutant Huntingtin PET Radioligands ^{11}C CHDI-00485180-R and ^{11}C CHDI-00485626 2023 [updated January. Available from: https://ClinicalTrials.gov/show/NCT03810898

[222] Mason SL, Daws RE, Soreq E, Johnson EB, Scahill RI, Tabrizi SJ, et al. Predicting clinical diagnosis in Huntington's disease: An imaging polymarker. Annals of Neurology. 2018;**83**(3):532-543

[223] Rizk-Jackson A, Stoffers D, Sheldon S, Kuperman J, Dale A, Goldstein J, et al. Evaluating imaging biomarkers for neurodegeneration in pre-symptomatic Huntington's disease using machine learning techniques. NeuroImage. 2011;**56**(2):788-796

[224] Mohan A, Sun Z, Ghosh S, Li Y, Sathe S, Hu J, et al. A machine-learning derived Huntington's disease progression model: Insights for clinical trial design. Movement Disorders. 2021. DOI: 10.1002/mds.28866

[225] Tan B, Shishegar R, Poudel GR, Fornito A, Georgiou-Karistianis N. Cortical morphometry and neural dysfunction in Huntington's disease: A review. European Journal of Neurology. 2020;**28**(4):1406-1419

Section 2

Advances in Treatment of Huntington's Disease

Chapter 5

Endocannabinoid System as a New Therapeutic Avenue for the Treatment of Huntington's Disease

Kamila Saramak and Natalia Szejko

Abstract

Huntington's disease (HD) is a progressive, neurodegenerative disorder manifested by chorea as well as a variety of psychiatric abnormalities. Up to this date, only symptomatic treatment exists. Therefore, there is an urgent need for further therapies. Several neuroanatomical circuits are involved in the pathophysiology of HD, mainly the dopaminergic system. Animal studies and limited studies in humans have shown that abnormalities in the endocannabinoid system could also play an important role in the pathophysiology of HD. These findings have important clinical implications since cannabis-based medicines could potentially be used in the treatment of HD. The aim of this chapter is to summarize the current state of the research regarding the involvement of the endocannabinoid system in HD.

Keywords: chorea, Huntington's disease, experimental therapies, cannabis-based medicine, dronabinol

1. Introduction

Huntington's disease (HD) is a neurodegenerative disorder characterized by progressive motor dysfunction, cognitive decline as well as psychiatric disturbance [1, 2]. The prevalence of HD is estimated to be between 0.4 and 5.70 per 100,000. Since HD is a genetic disorder, the prevalence depends strongly on the study population and it is higher in Europe, North America, and Australia than in Asia [3]. HD is caused by a dominantly inherited CAG repeat expansion in the huntingtin gene (HTT). The disease develops in individuals bearing a number of repetitions greater than 40, whereby greater CAG repeats found in the huntingtin gene are associated with early-onset forms of the disorder, fast rate of disease progression, and the most severe neurological deficits [4].

The mean age of HD onset is around 40 years, meanwhile the Juvenile Onset Huntington's Disease (JOHD), occurs in individuals bearing more than 60 CAG repeats, which usually starts at the age of 21. HD eventually leads to death 15–20 years after the symptomatic onset [5]. It is believed that mutant huntingtin (mHTT) affects many cellular functions and leads to cell death, preferentially subpopulations of GABAergic medium spiny projection neurons and neurons in the cerebral cortex [1, 6]. This leads to imbalances in diverse neurotransmission, including the dopaminergic

(DA) and glutaminergic systems. In the early stages of HD, DA neurotransmission is increased, whereas expression of DA receptors is reduced. However, in the course of the disease DA neurotransmission decreases. In turn, time-dependent abnormal DA neurotransmission affects glutamate receptor modulation, which may cause excitotoxicity [7, 8]. As DA plays a crucial role in the control of coordinated movements, motivation, and reward as well as cognitive function, alterations in DA balance in the striatum and provoke neurological and psychiatric symptoms of HD. The early stages of the disease are often characterized by chorea, followed by akinesia, while dystonia is more typical for the late stages [9]. Major non-motor symptoms include apathy and depression, anxiety, irritability, or aggressive behavior [9]. Impairment in cognitive functioning eventually ending in dementia, which has been mentioned by George Huntington in his first report, is another integral part of the disease [10]. Until today, there is no cure for HD, and treatment is only symptomatic, targeting mainly dopaminergic and glutaminergic systems [11].

2. Possible role of the endocannabinoid system in Huntington's disease

Over the last 30 years, the endocannabinoid system (ECS) has emerged as an important neuromodulatory system, which could be efficiently targeted in a number of neurological diseases, including HD [8, 12, 13]. The primary cannabinoid receptor subtypes are cannabinoid receptors type 1 (CB1) and type 2 (CB2). The CB1 receptor is a protein-coupled receptor, highly expressed in the central nervous system (CNS), particularly in the neocortex, hippocampus, basal ganglia, cerebellum, and brainstem. In addition to its CNS location, CB1 has also been identified in numerous peripheral tissues and cell types [14]. On the other hand, the CB2 receptor is expressed mainly outside CNS, predominantly in the immune system. However, it has also been identified in the CNS, especially in the glial cells and brainstem neurons [15, 16]. The abovementioned high distribution of the CB1 receptor in basal ganglia indicates an indispensable role of the ECS in the control of movements by inhibitory modulation of other neurotransmitter systems [16]. Moreover, the CB1 receptors regulate glutamatergic neurotransmission under both physiological and pathological conditions and thus are able to downregulate excitotoxic glutamate release [17].

3. Studies in animal models

Studies in animal models suggest that the pathogenesis of HD may be related to an early and widespread reduction in the ECS, particularly to the loss of CB1 receptors [16, 18, 19] and decreased endocannabinoid levels in the striatum, which in turn may lead to hyperkinesia [19]. The administration of substances, which increase endocannabinoid activity led to a significant improvement of motor disturbances in a rat model of HD [16, 20]. In particular, Lastres-Becker et al. [17] hypothesized that substances that increase the endocannabinoid activity could be applied for the treatment of hyperkinetic symptoms. To test this hypothesis the authors created a rat model of HD through bilateral striatal injections of 3-nitropionic acid that leads to impaired striatal GABAergic neurotransmission. As a result, these rats started suffering from abnormal movements followed by motor depression. In addition, they demonstrated that the severity of motor hyperkinesias was correlated with decreased concentration of several neurotransmitters, such as GABA, dopamine, and their metabolites. Moreover, mRNA levels for the CB1 receptor were depleted in the caudate-putamen of 3-nitropropionic acid (3-NP) injected rats. In addition, the authors demonstrated a reduction in CB1 receptor binding in the caudate-putamen, the globus pallidus, and also substantia nigra. Finally, the administration of AM404, an inhibitor of endocannabinoid uptake, led to the alleviation of motor disturbances. The same group from Madrid [21] explored the status of CB1 receptors in the HD94 transgenic mouse model of HD. To investigate this problem, the authors analyzed mRNA levels of the CB1 receptor and the number of specific binding sites, and the activation of GTP-binding proteins by the CB1 receptor agonist. As a result, they have demonstrated that mRNA transcripts of the CB1 receptor were significantly decreased in selected regions of the brain, such as caudate in the HD transgenic mice compared to controls. This depletion was correlated with a marked reduction of reception density in the caudate, globus pallidus, and substantia nigra pars reticulata. In addition, the efficacy of CB1 receptor activation was depleted in the globus pallidus and there was a trend toward a decrease in substantia nigra.

Another significant contribution was done by the group from the Autonomous University in Madrid led by Isabel Lastres-Becker [22]. The scientists used a previously mentioned rat model of HD for this purpose created via bilateral intrastriatal injections of 3-NP. As a result, CB1 receptor binding and activation of GTP-binding proteins were also reduced in the basal ganglia. In parallel, the authors demonstrated a significant decrease of two endocannabinoids, anandamide and 2-arachidonoyl-glycerol in the striatum of affected rats, while there was an increase in anandamide concentration in the substantia nigra. Importantly, both CB1 receptors concentration, as well as endocannabinoid levels, were not changed in the cerebral cortex. Another study by the same group [23] has shown that compounds acting at the endocannabinoid systems reduce hyperkinesia in a rat model of HD. In particular, they applied AM404, an inhibitor of the endocannabinoid reuptake, which was able to reduce hyperkinesia and provoke recovery from neurochemical deficits.

As for exocannabinoids used in the treatment of neurological and psychiatric disorders, in one study [24], delta9-tetrahydrocannabinol (THC), a nonselective cannabinoid receptor agonist, and SR141716, a selective antagonist for the CB1 receptor, were tested in an animal model of HD. Surprisingly enough, the administration of THC increased malonate-induced striatal lesions, but SR141716 enhanced the same effect to an even greater extent. Another study examined the long-term effects of exocannabinoid exposure in animal models of HD. In this case, they used transgenic mice R6/1 of HD and administered THC for 8 weeks. This chronic treatment preserved CB1 receptors in the R6/1 striatum, suggesting that the manipulation of endocannabinoid levels warrants further exploration.

Similarly, Sagredo et al. [25] examined the neuroprotective effect of cannabinoids in rats with 3NP striatal lesions. To tackle this question, the authors used the CB1 agonist arachidonyl-2-chloroethylamide (ACEA), the CB2 agonist HU-308, and cannabidiol (CBD). Interestingly enough, the application of CBD, but not ACEA or HU-308 reversed the effects of 3NP. In particular, CBD reversed 3NP-induced reductions in GABA contents and mRNA levels of substance P (SP), neuronal-specific enolase (NSE), and superoxide dismutase-2 (SOD-2). The authors concluded that CBD has neuroprotective values, but mainly on striatal neurons projecting to substantia nigra. This neuroprotective effect was not reversed by the CB1 receptor antagonist SR141716. Pintor et al. [26] demonstrated that the cannabinoid receptor agonist, WIN 55,212–2, attenuates the effects induced by quinolinic acid (QA) in the rat striatum. In this study,

Reference	Model	Substance	Outcome
Lastres-Becker et al. [17]	3 NP rats	• AM404 (eCBRI)	AM404 reduced motor hyperactivity and improved toxin-induced GABA and dopamine deficits.
Lastres-Becker et al. [23]	3 NP rats	• AM404 (eCBRI) • VDM11 (eCBRI) • AM374 (inhibitor of endocannabinoid hydrolysis) • Capsaicin (VR1 agonist) • CP55,940 (CB1R and CB2R agonist)	AM404 reduced hyperkinesia in lesioned animals VDM11 and AM374 did not improve hyperkinesia. Capsaicin and CP55,940 reduced hyperkinesia. Capsaicin improved GABA and dopamine deficits in basal ganglia.
Lastres-Becker et al. [24]	Malonate rats	• THC • SR141716A (CB1R antagonist)	Exacerbation of neurotoxicity.
Lastres-Becker et al. [36]	3NP rats	• THC	Neuroprotection.
De Lago et al. [21]	3 NP rats	• Arvanil (eCBRI, CB1R and TRPV1 agonist)	Arvanil showed anti-hyperkinetic effects and increased the content of glutamate in the globus pallidus.
Pintor et al. [26]	Quinolinic acid rats	• WIN55,212-2 (CB1R and CB2R agonist) • AM-251 (CB1R antagonist)	WIN55,212-2 showed neuroprotective effects and AM-251 reversed them.
De Lago et al. [30]	Malonate rats	• UCM707 (eCBRI)	Reduction of hyperkinetic activity and increase both glutamate and GABA levels in the globus pallidus. No neuroprotection.
Sagredo et al. [25]	3 NP rats	• CBD	Neuroprotection.
Sagredo et al. [28]	1. Malonate mice 2. CB2R knockout mice	• HU-308 (CB2R agonist) • SR144528 (CB2R antagonist) • CBD • ACEA (CB1R agonist)	HU-308 was neuroprotective and reduced proinflammatory markers (TNF-alpha). These effects were reversed by SR144528. CBD and ACEA were not neuroprotective.
Palazuelos et al. [35]	Mice expressing mHTT or quinolinic acid exposure	• HU-308	HU-308 reduced quinolinic acid neurotoxicity.
Sotter et al. [34]	Pheochromocytoma cells expressing mHHT	• HU210 (CB1R and CB2R agonist)	HU210 caused small, but significant increase of cell survival. It excerted potentially toxic effects including increased huntingtin aggregation.

Reference	Model	Substance	Outcome
Dowie et al. [37]	R6/1 transgenic mice	• HU210 • THC	HU210 and THC did not improve motor symptoms. HU210 treatment was associated with seizures.
Valdeolivas S et al. [27]	Malonate rats	• THC/CBD • SR141716A • AM630 (CB2R antagonist)	THC/CBD was neuroprotective. SR141716 and AM630 reduced its neuroprotective effects

HD: Huntington disease; CB1R: cannabinoid receptor type 1; CB2R: cannabinoid receptor type 2; 3 NP mice: 3-nitropropionic acid; eCBRI: endocannabinoid re-uptake inhibitor; TRPV1: the transient receptor potential cation channel subfamily V member 1 (TrpV1); GABA: γ-aminobutyric acid; THC: tetrahydrocannabinol; CBD: cannabidiol; and ACEA: arachidonyl-2-chloroethylamide.

Table 1.
Studies investigating the relevance of endocannabinoid system in HD pathogenesis in animal models. Studies are presented in chronological order.

QA was introduced in the rat striatum and this, in turn, led to the reproduction of clinical features typical for HD. The administration of WIN 55,212–2 blocked the increase in extracellular glutamate induced by QA. During *in vivo* experiment, WIN 55,212–2 significantly improved the striatal damage induced by QA, but no effect was observed on a behavioral ground. Valdeolivas et al. [27] also explored the neuroprotective potential of cannabinoids in an experimental model of HD. In particular, they investigated *Sativex®*, a combination of tetrahydrocannabinol (THC) and CBD at a ratio of 1:1, to monitor the potential neuroprotective effects of cannabinoids. The authors applied both histological and biochemical markers. As a result, the application of malonate in the striatum led to an increase in edema, while *Sativex®* reduced it. Moreover, *Sativex®* led to a reduction in neurodegeneration and glial activation. Furthermore, the authors found that both CB1 and CB2 receptors are involved in the positive effects of cannabinoids on HD symptoms. Similar findings were reported by Sagredo et al. [28], who used an animal model of HD to examine the potential neuroprotective effects of compounds influencing the endocannabinoid system. Interestingly enough, only compounds activating CB2 receptors had neuroprotective effects. The authors confirmed this statement by using the selective CB2 receptor antagonist, SR144528, which, in turn, led to increased vulnerability to malonate. What is more, the activation of CB2 receptors reduced the levels of tumor necrosis factor-alpha (TNF-alpha) that had been increased in the malonate-induced model of HD.

Another study by de Lago et al. [29] examined whether arvanil, an endocannabinoid „hybrid," could lead to symptom reduction in the rat model of HD. It was demonstrated that arvanil reduced ambulation and stereotypic movements. The same group [30] demonstrated that UCM707, an inhibitor of the anandamide uptake, could be used as a symptom control agent in an animal model of HD and multiple sclerosis (MS), but failed to delay the disease progression.

Furthermore, a number of other studies have suggested that therapies with CB-activating compounds might lead to neuroprotective effects against excitotoxic striatal toxicity through both CB receptor-mediated and independent effects [21, 31–35]. However, in several studies, no benefit or even exacerbation of neurotoxicity could be observed [22, 25, 29].

An overview of studies investigating the relevance of the endocannabinoid system in HD pathogenesis in animal models is shown in **Table 1**.

4. Clinical research

The post-mortem examination of brain tissue in individuals with HD as well as PET imaging studies *in vivo* showed that CB1 receptors are severely reduced in all regions of the basal ganglia in comparison to other receptor changes in HD, which strengthens the hypothesis of a possible role of cannabinoids in the progression of neurodegeneration in HD [38, 39].

First reports of using cannabinoids in patients with HD were contradictory [24, 28, 30]. In 1991, Consroe et al. conducted the first double-blind randomized cross-over study to evaluate the efficacy and safety of oral CBD (10 mg/kg/day for 6 weeks) in 15 neuroleptic-free patients with HD [28]. The therapeutic response was evaluated with the use of the Marsden and Quinn chorea severity scalc [40]. In this study, no statistically significant improvement has been shown. There was also no significant difference between the CBD and placebo groups in terms of side effects. In 1999 Müller-Vahl et al. published a case of a 58-year-old male with HD who was treated with a single dose of 1.5 mg of a CB1 agonist, nabilone. In this individual, a severe deterioration of chorea was observed [24]. In 2006, Curtis et al. described a case of a 43-year-old female, whose chorea and irritability improved after medication with 1 mg of nabilone [30]. A double-blind placebo-controlled randomized cross-over trial using nabilone was conducted in 2009 by the same author. This time 37 patients were treated with 1 mg or 2 mg of nabilone daily for 5 weeks. For primary measures, the patients were assessed with Unified Huntington's Disease Rating Scale (UHDRS) total motor score and

Reference	Number of patients (sex)	Age (mean)	Substance	Study design	Outcome
Consroe et al. [41]	15 (8 male, 7 female)	No data	CBD	Double-blind, randomized cross-over study	No significant improvement No relevant side effects
Müller-Vahl et al. [42]	1 male	58	Nabilone	Case report	Deterioration of chorea
Curtis et al. [43]	1 female	43	Nabilone	Case report	Improvement of chorea and irritability
Curtis et al. [44]	44 (22 male, 22 female)	52	Nabilone	Double-blind, placebo-controlled, cross-over study	Improvement of the UHDRS-chorea; 1 SAE – sedation
Moreno et al. [45]	25 (14 male, 11 female)	47.6	Nabiximols	Double-blind, randomized, cross-over, placebo-controlled, pilot trial	No SAE or clinical worsening; no significant improvement; no significant changes of biomarkers

CBM: cannabis based medicine; HD: Huntington disease; SAE: severe adverse events; CBD: cannabidiol; UHDRS: United Huntington Disease Rating Scale; and SAE: serious adverse events.

Table 2.
An overview of studies investigating efficacy and safety of CBM in HD.

UHDRS subsections for chorea, cognition and behavior, and neuropsychiatric inventory (NPI) for secondary measures. There were no statistically significant differences in total UHDRS between the groups. However, statistically, significant improvements were noted for the UHDRS chorea scale and the neuropsychiatric inventory. There were no statistical differences reported between the 1 and 2 mg. Adverse effects were reported for placebo and nabilone similarly. There was one Serious Adverse Event (SAE) related to nabilone—one of the patients withdrew due to severe sedation. Importantly, no psychoses were reported [23]. In 2016, the results of a study conducted by Moreno et al. using nabiximols in the treatment of HD were published [36]. Nabiximols (tradename *Sativex®*) is an oromucosal spray, containing 2.7 mg THC and 2.5 mg cannabidiol (CBD) per puff licensed in most European countries for symptomatic treatment of multiple sclerosis [35]. Both Sativex and placebo were handed to 25 patients in a form of an oral spray, to be administered up to 12 sprays/day for 12 weeks. The main aim of the study was to investigate the safety of nabiximols in HD patients, assessed by the absence of SAE and lack of impairment of motor, cognitive, behavioral, and functional scales during the active treatment. The secondary objective was a clinical improvement of Unified Huntington Disease Rating Scale scores. As a result, safety and tolerability were confirmed. No statistically significant improvement in UHDRS in the nabiximols group was noted with respect to the placebo group. Moreover, no significant changes in the biomarkers could be observed [35].

An overview of all available studies investigating the efficacy and safety of CBM in HD is provided in **Table 2**.

5. Safety profile of cannabis-based medicines in patients with HD

Even today, very little is known about the safety of CBM in patients with HD due to the limited number of studies exploring this issue. However, the available preliminary results suggest that the safety profile of CBM in HD is similar to that in other groups of patients. A recently conducted meta-analysis, including diverse populations of patients treated with CBM, showed that administration of cannabinoids can be associated with a greater risk of adverse events (AE), including serious adverse events (SAE) [46]. The most common short-term AEs included dizziness, dry mouth, nausea or vomiting, fatigue, somnolence, euphoria, vomiting, disorientation, drowsiness, confusion, loss of balance, and hallucinations. So far, there has been no study evaluating the long-term AEs of cannabinoids [46]. Up to this point, only two CBM-related SAEs in HD have been reported and both occurred after the treatment with nabilone. A 58-year-old male described by Müller-Vahl experienced an exacerbation of chorea. Moreover, the patient noticed the deterioration of short-term memory [42]. During the study performed by Curtis et al. [44], one of the patients experienced severe sedation and had to withdraw from the trial. Importantly, none of the patients enrolled in this study suffered from exacerbation of chorea or psychosis. The most frequent AE was drowsiness and forgetfulness. In the recent study conducted by Moreno et al. [45], dizziness or disturbance in attention were the two most common AEs. No serious alterations in psychiatric or neurological conditions of the participants were noted [45].

6. Conclusions

There is increasing evidence that the endocannabinoid system is a new promising therapeutical target in patients with HD. However, larger well-designed controlled studies are urgently needed to confirm the efficacy and safety of this treatment.

Author details

Kamila Saramak[1] and Natalia Szejko[2,3]*

1 Department of Neurology, Hochzirl Hospital, Zirl, Austria

2 Department of Bioethics, Medical University of Warsaw, Poland

3 Department of Neurology, Medical University of Warsaw, Warsaw, Poland

*Address all correspondence to: natalia.szejko@wum.edu.pl

References

[1] Ross CA, Tabrizi SJ. Huntington's disease: From molecular pathogenesis to clinical treatment. The Lancet Neurology. 2011;**10**:83-98

[2] Tabrizi SJ, Flower MD, Ross CA, Wild EJ. Huntington disease: New insights into molecular pathogenesis and therapeutic opportunities. Nature Reviews Neurology. 2020;**16**:529-546

[3] Pringsheim T, Wiltshire K, Day L, Dykeman J, Steeves T, Jette N. The incidence and prevalence of Huntington's disease: A systematic review and meta-analysis. Movement Disorders. 2012;**27**:1083-1091

[4] Walker FO. Huntington's disease. The Lancet. 2007;**369**:218-228

[5] Ribaï P, Nguyen K, Hahn-Barma V, Gourfinkel-An I, Vidailhet M, Legout A, et al. Psychiatric and cognitive difficulties as indicators of juvenile Huntington disease onset in 29 patients. Archives of Neurology. 2007;**64**:813-819

[6] Pazos M, Sagredo O, Fernandez-Ruiz J. The endocannabinoid system in Huntington's disease. Current Pharmaceutical Design. 2008;**14**:2317-2325

[7] Cepeda C, Murphy KP, Parent M, Levine MS. The role of dopamine in Huntington's disease. Progress in Brain Research. 2014;**211**:235-254

[8] Klein MO, Battagello DS, Cardoso AR, Hauser DN, Bittencourt JC, Correa RG. Dopamine: Functions, signaling, and association with neurological diseases. Cellular and Molecular Neurobiology. 2019;**39**:31-59

[9] van Duijn E, Craufurd D, Hubers AA, Giltay EJ, Bonelli R, Rickards H, et al. Neuropsychiatric symptoms in a European Huntington's disease cohort (REGISTRY). Journal of Neurology, Neurosurgery and Psychiatry. 2014;**85**:1411-1418

[10] Wexler A, Wild EJ, Tabrizi SJ. George Huntington: A legacy of inquiry, empathy and hope. Brain. 2016;**139**:2326-2333

[11] Bachoud-Lévi A-C, Ferreira J, Massart R, Youssov K, Rosser A, Busse M, et al. International guidelines for the treatment of Huntington's disease. Frontiers in Neurology. 2019;**10**:710

[12] Kluger B, Triolo P, Jones W, Jankovic J. The therapeutic potential of cannabinoids for movement disorders. Movement Disorders. 2015;**30**:313-327

[13] Szejko N, Saramak K, Lombroso A, Müller-Vahl K. Cannabis-based medicine in treatment of patients with Gilles de la Tourette syndrome. Neurologia i Neurochirurgia Polska. 2022;**56**:28-38

[14] Howlett A, Barth F, Bonner T, Cabral G, Casellas P, Devane W, et al. International Union of Pharmacology. XXVII. Classification of cannabinoid receptors. Pharmacological Reviews. 2002;**54**:161-202

[15] Van Sickle MD, Duncan M, Kingsley PJ, Mouihate A, Urbani P, Mackie K, et al. Identification and functional characterization of brainstem cannabinoid CB2 receptors. Science. 2005;**310**:329-332

[16] Jordan CJ, Xi Z-X. Progress in brain cannabinoid CB2 receptor research: From genes to behavior. Neuroscience and Biobehavioral Reviews. 2019;**98**:208-220

[17] Lastres-Becker I, Hansen HH, Berrendero F, De Miguel R, Pérez-Rosado A, Manzanares J, et al. Alleviation of motor hyperactivity and neurochemical deficits by endocannabinoid uptake inhibition in a rat model of Huntington's disease. Synapse. 2002;**44**:23-35

[18] Romero J, Lastres-Becker I, de Miguel R, Berrendero F, Ramos JA, Fernández-Ruiz J, et al. The endogenous cannabinoid system and the basal ganglia: Biochemical, pharmacological, and therapeutic aspects. Pharmacology. 2002;**95**:137-152

[19] Zlas J, Stark H, Seligman J, Levy R, Werker E, Breuer A, et al. Early medical use of cannabis. Nature. 1993;**363**:215

[20] Mechoulam R, Hanuš LO, Pertwee R, Howlett AC. Early phytocannabinoid chemistry to endocannabinoids and beyond. Nature Reviews Neuroscience. 2014;**15**:757-764

[21] Lastres-Becker I, Berrendero F, Lucas J, Martın-Aparicio E, Yamamoto A, Ramos J, et al. Loss of mRNA levels, binding and activation of GTP-binding proteins for cannabinoid CB1 receptors in the basal ganglia of a transgenic model of Huntington's disease. Brain Research. 2002;**929**:236-242

[22] Lastres-Becker I, Fezza F, Cebeira M, Bisogno T, Ramos JA, Milone A, et al. Changes in endocannabinoid transmission in the basal ganglia in a rat model of Huntington's disease. Neuroreport. 2001;**12**:2125-2129

[23] Lastres-Becker I, De Miguel R, De Petrocellis L, Makriyannis A, Di Marzo V, Fernández-Ruiz J. Compounds acting at the endocannabinoid and/or endovanilloid systems reduce hyperkinesia in a rat model of Huntington's disease. Journal of Neurochemistry. 2003;**84**:1097-1109

[24] Lastres-Becker I, Bizat N, Boyer F, Hantraye P, Brouillet E, Fernández-Ruiz J. Effects of cannabinoids in the rat model of Huntington's disease generated by an intrastriatal injection of malonate. Neuroreport. 2003;**14**:813-816

[25] Sagredo O, Ramos JA, Decio A, Mechoulam R, Fernández-Ruiz J. Cannabidiol reduced the striatal atrophy caused 3-nitropropionic acid in vivo by mechanisms independent of the activation of cannabinoid, vanilloid TRPV1 and adenosine A2A receptors. European Journal of Neuroscience. 2007;**26**:843-851

[26] Pintor A, Tebano M, Martire A, Grieco R, Galluzzo M, Scattoni M, et al. The cannabinoid receptor agonist WIN 55,212-2 attenuates the effects induced by quinolinic acid in the rat striatum. Neuropharmacology. 2006;**51**:1004-1012

[27] Valdeolivas S, Satta V, Pertwee RG, Fernández-Ruiz J, Sagredo O. Sativex-like combination of phytocannabinoids is neuroprotective in malonate-lesioned rats, an inflammatory model of Huntington's disease: Role of CB1 and CB2 receptors. ACS Chemical Neuroscience. 2012;**3**:400-406

[28] Sagredo O, González S, Aroyo I, Pazos MR, Benito C, Lastres-Becker I, et al. Cannabinoid CB2 receptor agonists protect the striatum against malonate toxicity: Relevance for Huntington's disease. Glia. 2009;**57**:1154-1167

[29] de Lago E, Urbani P, Ramos JA, Di Marzo V, Fernández-Ruiz J. Arvanil, a hybrid endocannabinoid and vanilloid compound, behaves as an antihyperkinetic agent in a rat model of Huntington's disease. Brain Research. 2005;**1050**:210-216

[30] De Lago E, Fernández-Ruiz J, Ortega-Gutiérrez S, Cabranes A,

Pryce G, Baker D, et al. UCM707, an inhibitor of the anandamide uptake, behaves as a symptom control agent in models of Huntington's disease and multiple sclerosis, but fails to delay/arrest the progression of different motor-related disorders. European Neuropsychopharmacology. 2006;**16**:7-18

[31] Pertwee RG. Cannabinoid pharmacology: The first 66 years. British Journal of Pharmacology. 2006;**147**:S163-SS71

[32] Pertwee RG. Emerging strategies for exploiting cannabinoid receptor agonists as medicines. British Journal of Pharmacology. 2009;**156**:397-411

[33] Collin C, Davies P, Mutiboko I, Ratcliffe S, Group SSiMS. Randomized controlled trial of cannabis-based medicine in spasticity caused by multiple sclerosis. European Journal of Neurology. 2007;**14**:290-296

[34] Scotter E, Goodfellow C, Graham E, Dragunow M, Glass M. Neuroprotective potential of CB1 receptor agonists in an in vitro model of Huntington's disease. British Journal of Pharmacology. 2010;**160**:747-761

[35] Palazuelos J, Aguado T, Pazos MR, Julien B, Carrasco C, Resel E, et al. Microglial CB2 cannabinoid receptors are neuroprotective in Huntington's disease excitotoxicity. Brain. 2009;**132**:3152-3164

[36] Lastres-Becker I, Bizat N, Boyer F, Hantraye P, Fernández-Ruiz J, Brouillet E. Potential involvement of cannabinoid receptors in 3-nitropropionic acid toxicity in vivo. Neuroreport. 2004;**15**:2375-2379

[37] Dowie M, Howard M, Nicholson L, Faull R, Hannan A, Glass M. Behavioural and molecular consequences of chronic cannabinoid treatment in Huntington's disease transgenic mice. Neuroscience. 2010;**170**:324-336

[38] Glass M, Dragunow M, Faull R. The pattern of neurodegeneration in Huntington's disease: A comparative study of cannabinoid, dopamine, adenosine and GABAA receptor alterations in the human basal ganglia in Huntington's disease. Neuroscience. 2000;**97**:505-519

[39] Van Laere K, Casteels C, Dhollander I, Goffin K, Grachev I, Bormans G, et al. Widespread decrease of type 1 cannabinoid receptor availability in Huntington disease in vivo. Journal of Nuclear Medicine. 2010;**51**:1413-1417

[40] Mestre TA, Forjaz MJ, Mahlknecht P, Cardoso F, Ferreira JJ, Reilmann R, et al. Rating scales for motor symptoms and signs in Huntington's disease: Critique and recommendations. Movement Disorders Clinical Practice. 2018;**5**:111-117

[41] Consroe P, Laguna J, Allender J, Snider S, Stern L, Sandyk R, et al. Controlled clinical trial of cannabidiol in Huntington's disease. Pharmacology Biochemistry. 1991;**40**:701-708

[42] Müller-Vahl KR, Schneider U, Emrich HM. Nabilone increases choreatic movements in Huntington's disease. Movement Disorders. 1999;**14**: 1038-1040

[43] Curtis A, Rickards H. Nabilone could treat chorea and irritability in Huntington's disease. The Journal of Neuropsychiatry. 2006;**18**:553-554

[44] Curtis A, Mitchell I, Patel S, Ives N, Rickards H. A pilot study using nabilone for symptomatic treatment in Huntington's disease. Movement Disorders. 2009;**24**:2254-2259

[45] Moreno JLL-S, Caldentey JG, Cubillo PT, Romero CR, Ribas GG, Arias MAA, et al. A double-blind, randomized, cross-over, placebo-controlled, pilot trial with Sativex in Huntington's disease. Journal of Neurology, Neurosurgery and Psychiatry. 2016;**263**:1390-1400

[46] Whiting PF, Wolff RF, Deshpande S, Di Nisio M, Duffy S, Hernandez AV, et al. Cannabinoids for medical use: A systematic review and meta-analysis. JAMA. 2015;**313**:2456-2473

Chapter 6

Advances in Cellular and Cell-Free Therapy Medicinal Products for Huntington Disease Treatment

Irina Kerkis, Rodrigo Pinheiro Araldi,
Cristiane Valverde Wenceslau and Thais Biude Mendes

Abstract

Huntington's disease (HD) is a neurodegenerative disorder caused by the expansion of CAG repeats in the huntingtin gene. The disease causes the progressive degeneration of neurons affecting particularly the medium spiny neurons (MSNs) within the striatum. The mHtt inclusions promote neurodegeneration. However, the mHtt can spread to different brain areas through exosomes. For this reason, it is not surprising that HD causes motor, cognitive and neuropsychiatric dysfunctions. To date there is no treatment able to modify the natural history of the disease. In this sense, the advanced cellular therapy, based on the therapeutic use of mesenchymal stem cells (MSCs) emerges as a potential candidate for HD treatment. This is because, the MSCs produce many critical therapeutic molecules which act in multiple cellular and molecular targets. Moreover, in addition, advanced cell therapy is a unique approach that could provides neuroprotection and neuroregeneration. However, the current discovery that the MSC mechanism of action is mediated by exosomes, have encouraged scientist to explore the therapeutic potential of the cell-free therapy. Based on this, we revisited the HD pathophysiology, areas. Providing evidence that MSC and MSC-derived exosomes can be used to change the natural history of HD.

Keywords: Huntington's disease, stem cells, therapeutic cells, exosomes, cell-free products

1. Introduction

Huntington's disease (HD, OMIM 143100) is a rare and incurable hereditary autosomal dominant neurodegenerative disorder, affecting 5–10 individuals per 100,000 in the Caucasian population. In certain regions, such as Australia, North America, and Western Europe, including the United Kingdom, the prevalence of the disease has increased over the past 50 years [1, 2].

HD is characterized by the loss of specific neurons within the striatum. The most sensitive cell population is the gamma-aminobutyric acid (GABA)ergic medium spiny neurons (MSNs). Neuropathologically, the disease leads to about 57% loss of cross-sectional area from the caudate nucleus and about 65% loss of the putamen (in *postmortem* samples). The progression of HD also leads to loss of cortical volume (particularly in cases with more advanced disease), affecting the large pyramidal neurons predominantly in layers III, V, and VI. In these cases, the loss of neurons in the thalamus, substantia nigra pars reticulata, and the subthalamic nucleus can also be observed. The neurodegeneration of these brain areas results in progressive motor (chorea, saccadic eye movement abnormalities, ataxia of speech, dysphagia, etc.), cognitive (dementia), and neuropsychiatric disturbances (depression, anxiety, apathy, etc.). These HD symptoms usually develop between ages 30 and 50 (adult-onset Huntington's disease—AOHD, which is verified in 95% of cases), but they can appear as early as age 20 (juvenile-onset Huntington's disease—JOHD). However, neurological loss and metabolic alterations generally occur in the adult HD brain before symptoms, but the precise timetable for the neuronal degeneration remains unknown [3].

HD is caused by the expansion of trinucleotide Cytosine-Adenine-Guanine (CAG) repeat, located in the first exon of the HD gene, also known as HTT or IT15 gene (locus 4p16.3, OMIM 613004), which encodes the huntingtin protein (Htt). Since the discovery of HTT gene mutation (in 1993), it has been recognized that larger CAG expansions are associated with early-onset in HD, especially for AOHD. Generally, unaffected individuals have less than 35 CAG repeats (common rage in humans: 17–25), while affected individuals have 36–250 CAG repeats. The CAG repeat range of 36–39 might be found in affected individuals and asymptomatic individuals (reduced penetrance alleles), whereas individuals with over 40 CAG repeats always develop the disease (fully penetrance alleles) [4].

The wild-type allele of the HTT gene (i.e., <35 CAG repeats) typically segregates and stably as a polymorphic locus. However, the allele carrying higher-normal CAG repeats (27–35 repeats) has increased instability. For this reason, individuals with 27–35 CAG repeats have a high risk of passing on repeats in the affected size range to their offspring. HTT gene encodes the huntingtin protein (Htt), a sizeable soluble protein (350 kDa), consisting of 3114 amino acids, which is expressed in all metazoans, is highly conserved among vertebrates. Although, all tissues ubiquitously express the HTT gene, Htt protein is found higher expressed in the brain, represented by all neurons and glial cells [4].

1.1 Htt protein characterization and function in HD

The Htt protein is crucial for developing and maintaining central nervous systems (CNS) homeostasis since the protein is engaged in many cellular and biological functions, including transcription, transport, vesicular trafficking, and coordination of cell division, energy metabolism, and antiapoptotic activity. For this reason, it is not surprised that Htt co-localizes with many organelles, such as the nucleus, endoplasmic reticulum, Golgi complex, endosomes, mitochondria, and synaptic vesicles. Furthermore, cells expressing mRNA of the HTT gene were described by in situ hybridization in the usual human 20 to 23-week fetal brain, suggesting that huntingtin protein is crucial for the development of the CNS. Studies also demonstrated that the deletion of the mouse homolog of the HTT gene is lethal in the embryo before the brain is formed. By contrast, heterozygote mice for the HTT gene usually develop but exhibit motor deficits and cell loss in basal ganglia. Altogether, these data confirm that the Htt protein is mandatory for CNS development and function [5].

The Htt protein is characterized by the presence of (i) the N-terminal 17 amino acids (or N17 region), which is followed by (ii) the polyglutamine (poly Q) tract (encoded by the CAG repeats), (iii) a proline-rich region (PRR), (iii) clusters of Huntingtin, Elongation factor 3, PR65/A regulatory subunit of PP2A and target of rapamycin 1 (HEAT) repeats (α-helix-loop-α-helix motif), and (iv) caspase and calpain cleavage sites (in higher vertebrates). The N17 region has been identified as a critical region that plays a role in Htt localization, aggregation, and toxicity. It is subject to several post-translational modifications, including acetylation, SUMOylation, phosphorylation, and ubiquitination. The polyQ tract is encoded by the CAG trinucleotide repeats, which code for the glutamine (Q) amino acid. PRP region is exclusively found in mammals and is essential for the Htt interactions with proteins containing tryptophans or Src homology 3 domains. In addition, PRP encodes the polyproline (polyP) region, which interacts with polyQ, increasing the Htt protein stability and solubility. HEAT repeats consist of around 50 amino acids and contains two antiparallel α-helices forming a hairpin, which acts as a scaffold for various protein complexes and mediates inter and intramolecular interactions. Sixteen HEAT repeats organized into four clusters were identified in the Htt protein. Htt protein also has several proteolytic cleavage sites, including proline, glutamic acid, serine, and threonine domains. These domains are found in both Htt and mHtt proteins. Thus, these proteins can be cleaved by caspase 3 at amino acid 513 and 552, caspase 1 at amino acid 572, caspase 2 at amino acid 552, and caspase 6 at position 586. In addition, two calpain cleavage sites are located at amino acid 469 and 536, and the metalloproteinase (MMP)-10 cleaves Htt our mHtt at amino acid 402 [5].

The Htt protein interacts with over 200 other proteins, many of them involved in microtubule-mediated axon traffickings, such as the Huntingtin-associated protein 1 (HAP1), which mediates the interaction between Htt protein with microtubule motor proteins and their co-factors (kinesin, dynactin subunit p150, and dynein). Htt protein also mediates long- and short-range axonal transport and vesicle trafficking. This is because the Htt protein binds to the endocytic pathway-related proteins (clathrin and dynamin), as well as endocytic organelle trafficking proteins (α-adaptin, Hip1, Hip14, HAP40, PACSIN1, SH3GL3/endophilin 3). Htt protein is enriched at synaptic terminals and interacts with cytoskeletal and synaptic vesicle proteins to regulate synaptic activity in neurons. However, by exhibiting a C-terminus containing a nuclear export signal (NES), Htt protein can traffics between cytoplasm and nucleus. In addition, the N17 region also interacts with a nuclear pore protein (TRP), which has nuclear translocation activity. The N-terminal domain also forms an amphipathic alpha-helical membrane-binding domain that reversibly mediates association with the endoplasmic reticulum (ER), endosomes, and autophagic vesicles. Thus, it is not surprising that Htt protein also interacts with various transcription factors and transcriptional regulatory proteins, acting as a positive regulator of brain-derived neurotrophic factor (BDNF) transcription (a protein in which expression levels are found reduced in individuals with HD), stimulating the BDNF vesicular trafficking in neurons.

However, by increasing the number of glutamine residues in poliQ, the CAG trinucleotide expansion, verified in HD, reduces the solubility of mutated huntingtin protein (mHtt), resulting in intracellular aggregates (inclusions) in the brain, particularly in GABAergic medium spiny neurons (MSNs), located within the striatum. This event occurs because the expanded polyQ sequence in mHtt protein undergoes conformational changes to form a B-pleated sheet prone to aggregation. In addition, the early phases of aggregate formation appear to accelerate the hydrophobic interactions with an amphipathic α-helical structure of N17. Under physiological conditions, proteostasis balances protein synthesis, folding, trafficking, and degradation. The impairment of the proteostasis systems aggravates the aggregation of the misfolded mHtt. In addition, posttranslational modifications influence the mHtt toxicity, aggregation propensity, and intracellular localization. For example, proteolytic cleavage of mHtt generates N-terminal fragments with an increased tendency to aggregate. Furthermore, the mHtt inclusions can block the axonal transport between the cell body and the synaptic cleft and recruit other polyQ-containing proteins, which interact with mHtt, leading to loss of biological function, therefore, cell death. In addition, mHtt also silences the activity of RE1-Silencing Transcription Factor (REST), increasing the binding of REST to RE1/neuron restrictive silencer element, producing transcriptional dysfunction [6, 7].

1.2 Htt protein and mitochondrial dysfunction

The mHtt inclusions promote mitochondrial dysfunction, decreasing the activity of mitochondrial respiratory complexes II, III, and IV, which was already verified in *postmortem* brain samples of HD patients. Furthermore, the activity decrease of these mitochondrial complexes was also reported in asymptomatic HD carriers, indicating that mitochondrial defects may initiate disease onset. Experimental results also demonstrated that the ectopic expression of mitochondrial complex II subunit in striatal neurons expressing mHtt exon 1 restores complex II respiratory activity and protects against cell death. Confirming this data, it was extensively demonstrated that the rats treated with the neurotoxin 3 -nitropropionic acid (3-NP)—a selective inhibitor of succinate dehydrogenase and complex II—recapitulates the loss of MSNs in the substantia nigra, resulting in HD-like symptoms. In addition, studies showed that humans exposed to 3-NP exhibit motor dysfunction similar to HD patients [8–11].

Moreover, the mHtt can be cleaved by caspase 6. The fragments of cleaved mHtt protein bind to several transcription regulators, including the tumor suppressor, p53, thus regulating genes involved in mitochondrial function. Therefore, the mHtt increased the levels of p53, which in turn increased Bax and Puma expression, resulting in mitochondrial dysfunction and neuronal loss. These actions increase the reactive oxygen species (ROS) production, justifying the oxidative damage commonly observed in the plasma of HD patients, HD *postmortem* brain tissue, lymphoblasts, and cerebrospinal fluid. In addition, markers of oxidative damage, including heme oxygenase (an inducible isoform that occurs in response to oxidative stress), 3-nitrotyrosine (a marker for peroxynitrite-mediated protein nitration), and malondialdehyde (MDA), are elevated in human HD striatum and cortex as compared with age-matched control brain specimens. Consistent with these data, an increase in 8-hydroxy-2′-deoxyguanosine (8-OHdG), a marker of oxidative DNA damage, in both plasma and urine of HD patients is observed [8–11].

Cumulative evidence has also demonstrated that mHtt protein causes a reduction in TORC1, the most potent transcriptional activator of (peroxisome proliferator-activated receptor (PPAR)-γ coactivator-1 (PCG-1α) [12–14]. In addition, the mHtt protein also increases transglutaminase (Tgase) activity, which impairs the transcription of PCG-1α. Thus, mHtt downregulates the expression levels of PCG-1α [14]. The last is recognized as a critical transcriptional coactivator, which interacts with a broad range of transcription factors within a variety of biological processes. In addition, PCG-1α is involved in the regulation of mitochondrial biogenesis, OXPHOS, antioxidant defense, adaptive thermogenesis, and glucose/fatty acid metabolism. Under physiological conditions, the PGC-1α forms heteromeric complexes with nuclear respiratory factors (NRF-1 and NRF-2), and with the nuclear receptors (PPARα, PPARδ, PPARγ and estrogen-related receptor α (ERRα)). These heterodimers regulate the expression of many nuclear-encoded mitochondrial genes, including cytochrome c, complexes I–V, and the mitochondrial transcription factor A (Tfam), as well as antioxidant genes, including superoxide dismutase (SOD) and glutathione peroxidase (GPX). Thus, the mitochondrial dysfunctions promoted by the mHtt-mediated PCG-1α downregulation lead to an increase in oxidative stress [12, 13, 15].

1.3 Htt protein and neuroinflammation

In addition, the mHtt accumulation in neurons promotes microglial activation, increasing oxidative stress. In addition, microglial cells that express mHtt show significant elevations in nuclear factor kappa B (NF-κB). This elevation occurs because the mHtt interacts with the IκB kinase (IKK) γ subunit, promoting the assembly and activation of the IKK complex (comprised by IKKα and IKKβ subunits). The IKKβ kinase phosphorylates IκBα causes the liberation of NF-κB, promotes the gene expression of the pro-inflammatory cytokine, including interleukin (IL)-6, resulting in neuroinflammation [16, 17]. The neuroinflammatory cytokines produced in response to mHtt protein accumulation leading to the activation of microglial cells considered the brain's resident immune cells. Under physiological conditions, i.e., in the absence of inflammatory stimulus, microglia are in a surveilling state, being responsible for maintaining synapses and synaptic plasticity. In addition, Microglia also facilitates the growth and development of surrounding neural networks by secreting neurotrophic factors, such as BDNF, nerve growth factor (NGF), and insulin-like growth factor (IGF-1) [18]. Moreover, significant evidence suggests the microglia promotes neurogenesis by phagocytosing apoptotic neural cells, facilitating the migration and differentiation of neural progenitor cells, and secreting soluble factors related to neurogenesis. However, microglia become activated upon detecting inflammatory stimuli, such as the increase in ROS or cytokine production [19]. When activated, microglia can adopt different polarization states, such as M1 and M2. Interestingly, microglia can alternate between these states. For this reason, recently, studies have suggested using M1/M2 terminology to categorize activated microglial cells. M1 microglia exhibit a proinflammatory phenotype, the significant initiators of innate and adaptive immunity in the brain. In addition, these cells elicit a phagocytic function and release cytotoxic factors, including nitric oxide and ROS. M2 microglia also carry out phagocytosis, but contrary to the role of M1 microglia, M2 microglia exhibit an anti-inflammatory phenotype, releasing anti-inflammatory cytokines such as interleukin (IL)-4, IL-13, and transforming growth factor-beta (TGF-β), which suppress inflammatory responses. The continued activation of microglia, stimulated by the inclusions of mHtt, prolonged the production of inflammatory mediators, resulting in chronic inflammation. The last is implicated in further tissue damage, justifying the microglia activation in striatal GABAergic neurons verified by Positron Emission Tomography (PET) in HD patients. Interestingly, studies based on PET also reported the presence of microglia activation in striatal GABAergic neurons in presymptomatic HD gene carriers, suggesting that microglial activation is an early characteristic of HD before symptom onset. However, the activation of microglia increases oxidative stress, resulting in both nuclear and mitochondrial DNA oxidative damages and protein and lipid oxidation. These damages lead to progressive cell death, particularly of MSN's [20, 21].

1.4 Subventricular zone involvement in HD physiopathology

Studies based on animal models of HD demonstrate that cell death in the striatum serves as a potent stimulator of progenitor cell proliferation (which are resident into the subventricular zone – SVZ), neuroblast migration, and neurogenesis. This is because, in the transgenic mouse model of HD (in which there is minimal cell loss in the striatum), the SVZ is unaltered, while in rat striatal-lesion models of HD (in which there is a cell loss in the striatum), there is a marked increase in SVZ progenitor cell proliferation and neurogenesis. The SVZ of the lateral ventricle is the resident niche of stem cells. These stem cells give rise to proliferative progenitor cells during brain development, which migrates to the cortex or the basal ganglia, where they differentiate into neurons. SVZ preserves its critical developmental characteristics in the adult brain, responsible for the continuous generation of migrating neuroblasts destined for the olfactory bulb or other areas of cell death in the brain. Thus, the maintenance of SVZ is crucial for neuron replacement along adulthood [22–24].

Supporting the involvement of SVZ with the physiopathology of HD, several studies revealed that the SVZ of HD patients is enriched in endogenous factors and receptors that actively regulate the cell cycle and the differentiation of precursors, such as the neuropeptide Y. Furthermore, studies already showed a significant increase of GABAA, receptor subunit γ2 (involved in the desensitization of the receptor complex to GABA) in SVZ in HD. GABA is an essential trophic factor for neurons during development. High levels of GABA are found in the normal SVZ and the SVZ of HD patients, suggesting that the SVZ maintains a germinal capacity for proliferation and neurogenesis in response to neurodegenerative cell death in adult life. However, it was proved that, while the Htt protein interacts with cAMP response element-binding protein (CREB) and specificity proetin1 (Sp1), conferring anti-apoptotic action, the mHtt protein triggers a pathogenic cascade involving Sp1 transcription factor activation, which leads to repressor element-1 silencing transcription factor (REST) upregulation, repressing neuronal genes [22–24].

2. Exosomes

With the progression of HD, others brain areas, besides the substantia nigra, are subjected to neuronal loss, leading to cognitive and neuropsychiatric dysfunctions. This occurs because the mHtt (as the Htt) is widespread to different brain areas through extracellular vesicles (EVs). The EVs comprise a heterogeneous group of phospholipid bilayer-enveloped particles that are naturally produced and secreted into the extracellular environment by almost all cell types. According to their size, biogenesis, and content, these vesicles are classified as (i) microvesicles, (ii) exosomes, and (iii) apoptotic bodies. Among these vesicles, exosomes are the most investigated. This is because, due to the repertoire of bioactive molecules carried by these vesicles (coding and non-coding RNA, proteins, lipids, and metabolites), the exosomes play an important role in cell-to-cell communication and intercellular signaling, regulating both physiological and pathophysiological processes. Moreover, in the function of their nanosize (30–200 nm), exosomes easily cross the blood-brain barrier [1, 25].

The growing interest in this class of EV has been reflected in the creation of distinct databases that compile data on exosome content, such as Exocarta (http://www.exocarta.org/), EVpedia (http://bigd.big.ac.cn/databasecommons/database/

id/4354) and Vesiclepedia (http://microvesicles.org/), which are constantly updated with released studies.

Exosomes are formed by endocytosis and released by exocytosis. During the biogenesis of these vesicles, the inward budding of the plasma membrane results in small intracellular vesicles. These small vesicles fuse, forming early endosomes. The invagination of the early endosome membrane results in the formation of intraluminal vesicles (ILVs) within large multivesicular bodies (MVBs). In contrast, cytoplasmic molecules such as coding and non-coding RNA, proteins, lipids, and metabolites are engulfed and enclosed into the ILV lumen. Along with the maturation of early endosomes to late endosomes, some proteins are directly integrated into the invaginating membrane. However, this process depends on the endosomal sorting complexes required for transport (ESCRTs), which are comprised of four proteins (ESCRT-0, ESCRT-I, ESCRT-II, and ESCRT-III) that work cooperatively to facilitate the MVB formation, vesicle budding, and protein cargo sorting [1, 25]. The exosomes biogenesis also occurs through an ESCRT-independent pathway mediated by tetraspanins and ceramide-enriched lipid rafts. Tetraspanins are recruited at early steps to endosome membranes before ILV formation, and at least CD9, CD63, CD81, and CD82 are found in endosome and exosome membranes [1, 25].

Ceramides and their derived metabolites are organized in raft-based microdomains that interact with proteins, such as flotillins. The lipid-enriched structures are involved not only in endosomal membrane invagination for ILV formation but also in cargo loading. The selective cargo loading occurs during exosome biogenesis through tetraspanins-dependent and/or ESCRT-dependent mechanisms [1, 25]. Although, the biological cargo of exosomes varies widely according to their cell type of origin, they mainly consist of proteins, nucleic acids (particularly RNA) and lipids. More than 2400 different RNAs and, 4000 proteins were already identified and characterized in exosomes [1, 25].

Due to their endosomal origin, the exosomes are enriched in several proteins engaged in the biogenesis of MVBs, including clathrin, which can bind to hunting protein. Moreover, exosomes contain CD9, CD63, CD81, CD82, CD54, and CD11b tetraspanins, which serve as specific molecules. In addition, the exosomes contain heat shock proteins (HSP90, HSP70, and HSP60), which act as chaperones and play an essential role in cellular responses related to environmental stress. Besides this, exosomes also carry mRNA and a multitude of long non-coding (lnc) RNA and small RNA (particularly miRNA) that can be transferred into recipient cells, inducing cellular responses [1, 25–27].

The interaction of MVBs with actin and microtubules is essential for their transport to the plasma membrane. The translocation of MVB toward the plasma membrane depends on several molecules via the cytoskeleton. Rab GTPases such as RAB11, RAB27A/B, and RAB35 are mediators of selective sorting of MVB to the plasma membrane and exosome release. The MVBs are decorated with tethering protein complexes, such as HOPS and SNAREs, that mediate the fusion of these vesicles with the plasma membrane, The presence of tetraspanins and lysosomal-associated membrane proteins LAMP1 and LAMP2 in late endosomes also facilitate the fusion of MVB with the plasma membrane [1, 25].

After secretion, the exosomes will dock into the membrane of the target cells and activate signaling events or be internalized through specific receptor-ligand interactions. The transmembrane proteins present in the surface of exosomes (tetraspanins) can be recognized by signaling receptors in the target cells, resulting in activation of transduction pathways and modulation of the intracellular process without entering the target cells. Exosomes can merge with the target cells' plasma membrane, releasing its cargo directly into the cytosol by a low pH-dependent mechanism. However, the main route for exosome uptake can occur by clathrin-mediated or caveolin-dependent endocytosis, and the presence of lipid rafts in the membrane facilitates the process [1, 25].

After internalization, exosomes are sorted into MVB with two possible fates: (i) to be released again to neighboring cells or (ii) to be degraded after fusion of LE/MVB with lysosomes [1, 25]. The uptake of exosomes by brain cells seems to be cell type-dependent. For instance, neurons and glial cells seem to uptake exosomes by clathrin-mediated endocytosis. Some neurons can also use specific receptors from the SNARE family, such as SNAP25, for exosome uptake. Interestingly, the uptake of exosomes seems to be a selective pathway. Exosomes derived from cortical neurons were primarily internalized by hippocampal neurons, whereas astrocytes and oligodendrocytes took up exosomes released by neuroblastoma cell line N2A. Exosomes derived from oligodendrocytes are mainly internalized by microglia but not by neurons or astrocytes. In addition, the uptake of exosomes was also more active in pre-synaptic regions, which might indicate that these vesicles use constitutive endocytosis processes at these regions for neuronal cell entrance [1, 25].

2.1 Exosomes as a key mediator of HD pathophysiology

Initially, exosomes were considered vehicles for the elimination of cellular components. However, current studies have provided evidence that exosomes play multiple physiological roles in the nervous system. Exosomes are released by neural cells, including neurons, astrocytes, microglia, and oligodendrocytes, playing essential physiological roles in neurogenesis, synaptic activity and plasticity, myelination, and protection and regeneration neurons after injury and disease. Thus, it is not surprising that exosomes mediate the pathogenesis of neurodegenerative disorders, such as HD. This is because the misfolded proteins related to these disorders can be selectively integrated into ILVs of MVBs, and subsequently released into the extracellular environment within exosomes [28].

In HD, cumulative evidence has demonstrated that exosomes are implicated in the physiopathology of HD, serving as a vehicle for the expanded polyglutamine tract of HTT RNA and protein (mHtt), as well as mHtt aggregates transport to different brain areas. Supporting this evidence, it was verified that exosomes could deliver expanded trinucleotide repeat RNAs among cells and facilitate the propagation of mHtt protein [29–32]. It was shown that the injection of fibroblast-derived exosomes from an HD patient into a newborn mouse brain ventricles triggered the manifestation of HD-related behavior and pathology [31]. Moreover, it is known that the Htt protein regulates anterograde and retrograde transport of endocytic vesicles by interacting with several mediators, such as α-adaptin, Hip1, Hip14, HAP1, HAP40, SH3GL3, clathrin, and dynamin [29, 30]. This process is coordinated by the phosphorylation of Htt, which serves as a molecular decision marker for the anterograde or retrograde direction of vesicle transport. Thus, while the Htt promotes axonal BDNF vesicle trafficking, mHtt interacts with HIP1 and dynactin, leading to de-railing of molecular motors from microtubules tracks and cessation of transport [33].

3. Animal models for Huntington's disease

Animal models for HD have been successfully used for more than three decades to identify pathways involved in HD pathology or for preclinical testing of therapeutic strategies. These models are divided into (i) monogenetic and (ii) genetic murine models. However, none of these models can mimic the main feature of HD since no rodent model develops the chorea. For this reason, herein, we summarize the pros and cons of each animal model, considering their utility for preclinical test purposes [34–36].

3.1 Monogenetic models

Historically, monogenetic models have dominated the field of HD disease. These models are based on the use of toxins that typically induce cell death either by excitotoxic mechanism or by disruption of mitochondrial machinery. Among the excitotoxicity toxins used to obtain murine models for HD are quinolinic acid (QA) and kainic acid (KA). These neurotoxins induce cell death by binding to their cognate receptors, N-methyl-D-aspartic acid (NMDA) and non-NMDA, respectively, on striatal neurons. The QA or KA rat models exhibits motors (hyperkinesia, apomorphine-induced dystonia, and dyskinesia) and cognitive symptoms of HD (visuospatial deficits, procedural memory deficits, and poor memory recall). However, for various reasons, QA became the preferred excitotoxin for use in HD studies. The QA is formed from the metabolism of tryptophan via the kynurenine pathway, which is found in high quantities in the urine of rats that received a diet high in tryptophan. Interestingly, the tryptophan crosses the blood-brain barrier (BBB) using transporters shared by other neutral amino acids. In the brain, tryptophan is taken up by astrocytes, macrophages, microglia, and dendric cells and converted into kynurenine. In the presence of the enzymatic 3-hydroxyanthranilic acid oxygenase, a series of enzymatic reactions converts kynurenine to QA. Thus, the expected level of QA does not cause damage, but only small increases in QA levels cause toxicity. Moreover, it was verified that the administration of QA in the mouse models promotes the upregulation of Htt protein, linking the levels of this neurotoxin with HD pathogenesis. However, the QA is incapable of crossing the BBB. For this reason, the QA has been administrated directly within the brain [37–39].

Unlike the QA, the mitochondrial toxin 3-nitropropionic acid (3-NP) crosses the BBB and could be systemically administrated through intraperitoneal or subcutaneous injection [40–42].

The 3-NP is a plant (Indigofera endecapylla) and fungal (Aspergillus flavus, Astragalus, Arthrinium) toxin, which acts as an irreversible inhibitor of succinate dehydrogenase. It inhibits both the Krebs cycle and the mitochondrial complex II of the electron transport chain. The toxin also induces caspase-9 activation, which in turn requires the simultaneous presence of Apaf-1, cytochrome c, and ATP, suggesting that neuronal death may occur in the presence of intense ATP depletion. Moreover, the 3-NP induces oxidative and nitrate stress due to excessive ROS/RNS production and lack of the antioxidant system [40, 43–45]. Interesting, numerous studies demonstrated that the chronic systemic administration of 3-NP in rats impairs energy metabolism and results in striatal lesions, inducing a spectrum of HD-like pathology in rat striatum. In addition, in 1993, Beal et al. [41] showed that the 3-NP model causes selective striatal lesions characterized by the loss of medium spiny neurons (MSNs) and astroglial proliferation, replicating the histological and neurochemical features of HD. Although, the loss of MSNs in 3-NP rat models causes motor and cognitive symptoms analogous to those verified in HD, this model does not exhibit chorea.

However, the 3-NP model is capable of mimicking both hyperkinetic and hypokinetic symptoms of HD depending on the time course of administration. Thus, while the administration of 3-NP in two individual doses causes hyperkinetic movements analogous to those observed in early to mid-stage HD, the administration of more than four injections of 3-NP causes hypokinetic movements similar to those that appear in late-stage HD [40, 43–45]. Nevertheless, the response to the 3-NP changes according to the murine (CD1, C57BL/6, BALB/c, Sebster/Swiss and 129sEMS) or rat strain (Fischer, Lewis, and Wistar). In this sense, it is recognized that rats are most vulnerable to the toxic action of 3-NP treatment than mice. Fisher rats are the most susceptible to the 3-NP toxin but display significant variability in response to the toxin due to the difficulty of controlling damage caused by this toxin. In contrast, Lewis rats are less susceptible to 3-NP but respond more stably and consistently to 3-NP in behavioral alterations and lesions. Wistar and Sprague-Dawley rats are also sensitive to the 3-NP, developing lesions and behavioral modifications of extraordinary value for studying possible routes involved in HD and testing new therapeutic strategies. Although, the 3-NP model leads to a (i) massive cell death induced by the toxin, (ii) serving as a helpful model for (ii) analyzing and studying neuroprotective and (iii) neurorestorative therapies for HD patients, (iv) allowing to study the mechanisms involved in HD pathogenesis, including energy deregulations and ROS production, this model does not express the mHtt protein.

3.2 Genetic models

The genetic or transgenic animal models emerge as an alternative to nongenetic models since they express the mHtt protein [46, 47]. Transgenic models are divided into (i) those expressing transgenes with a truncated section of human HTT carrying the CAG repeats or full-length human HTT gene, and (ii) those with long CAG repeats replacing mouse Htt. Instability of the CAG repeat has been observed in many of the mouse models and was noted in the first HD model (R6 series). Although, different rodent models have been used to understand the biology of HD or employed in preclinical trials to investigate the therapeutic potential of products candidates to alleviate HD symptoms, they are limited in their ability to provide evidence of the effects of genetic modifiers of disease. In addition, there are many differences among the transgenic rodent models that can lead to different results, especially for preclinical trials.

In this sense, in two independent studies, it was demonstrated that a version of the R6/2 mouse with 90 CAG repeats (R6/2(CAG)90) shows earlier mHtt nuclear aggregation when compared to the R6/2 mouse with 200 CAG repeats (R6/2(CAG)200). Moreover, the R6/2(CAG)90 brains contain nuclear aggregates with a diffuse punctate appearance which remained partly detergent soluble, which correlated with the onset of transcriptional changes. In contrast, the R6/2(CAG)200 brains contain cytoplasmic aggregates that gave larger inclusion bodies related to behavioral changes. These data indicate that CAG length gives different phenotypes [48–50].

Several models encoding glutamine but using a mixed CAACAG rather than a pure CAG tract were developed to prevent germline and somatic expansion of CAG trinucleotide. An example of these models is the BACHD models with 97 glutamines encoded by a diverse CAACAG tract. These mice have five copies of the transgene integrated into their genome and express BACHD HTT, an estimated three-fold level of the transcript, and 1.5 to 2-fold protein level (mHtt).

BACHD rats show string impairment in muscle endurance at 2 months of age. Altered circadian rhythmic and locomotor activity are also observed in these animals [51–53]. However, the BACHD model is not commercially available, difficult to access this model.

4. Therapeutic cells: perspectives of HD treatment

When discovered, stem cells—therapeutic cells gain exceptional attention due to their capacity to produce precursors and differentiated cells. Propose, therefore, was to use stem cells in tissue regeneration [26, 27]. Stem cells showed differentiation potential *in vitro* and *in vivo* (animal models). Thus, we know two principal types of stem cells: adult and pluripotent. Pluripotent cells are embryonic stem cells or induced pluripotent stem cells, which are adult stem cells reversed in stem cells similar to embryonic [28]. However, this chapter will focus on adult stem cells isolated from different tissues like bone marrow, adipose tissue, umbilical cord, and dental pulp. Adult stem cells, especially mesenchymal stem cells (MSC), differ from their pluripotent counterparts, and being more mature, they cannot differentiate *in vivo* into appropriate tissue. However, these cells present specific characteristics that are of great interest in treating neurodegenerative diseases.

MSC secretes a large number of biologically active molecules, growth factors, hormones, interleukins, etc. [29]. These biomolecules can be found in free form or contained in exosomes, which are recognized as a key component in paracrine regulation [1, 25]. These molecules provide beneficial effects on injured tissues. For example, they induce angiogenesis and tissue regeneration and inhibit fibrosis, apoptosis, and inflammation [30–32]. In addition, which is essential for HD disease, MSCs and MSC's secretomes provide neurogenic, neuroprotective, and synaptogenic effects [33]. They improve the abnormal dopamine transmission and inflammatory reaction in the transgenic HD model [34]. Animal models showed that they produce factors protecting retinal ganglion cells against glutamate excitotoxicity, neurotrophins expressed by MSCs inhibit pro-inflammatory cytokine secretion, MSCs fight oxidative stress and others [35, 36]. Due to the characteristics above, MSCs called medicinal signaling cells or simply therapeutic cells [37].

4.1 Therapeutic cells

Medicinal signaling cells (MSC) have been used in a variety of preclinical studies, which were focused on behavioral and memory outcomes, reduction of brain damage and minimization of striatal degeneration. "Native" MSC isolated from different adult tissues such as bone marrow, adipose tissue and umbilical cord were used in these studies. Due to their ability to adhere to plastic, MSC can be easily isolated and expanded *in vitro* [38]. They are isolated and cultured using similar protocols and culture medium reagents. However, different research groups usually introduce a few modifications in the protocol, which may affect the MSC quality and efficiency. MSC can differentiate *in vitro*, especially into mesoderm derivatives, but not *in vivo*. After isolation, these cells express similar markers and share similar morphological features. However, different MSC populations can be isolated from the same or different tissues. These populations differ in self-renewal, plasticity and therapeutic potential [29, 39, 40]. To standardize the concept of MSC used in different studies and by various scientific groups the International Society for Gene and Cell Therapy (ISGCT) established the minimum criteria for defining these cells and populations isolated [41]. Despite MSC populations' heterogeneity, these cells share regenerative, anti-apoptotic, anti-fibrotic anti-inflammatory, immunosuppressive, immunomodulatory, and angiogenic properties [42].

4.2 Therapeutic cells in preclinical HD studies

Stem cell-based therapies are important to reconstruct damaged brain areas in HD patients. These therapies have a dual role: stem cell paracrine action, stimulating local cell survival, and brain tissue regeneration through the production of new neurons from the intrinsic and likely from donor stem cells. Initially, preclinical studies were mainly focused on the neuroprotective function of MSC. Since these cells express a variety of neurotrophins and in particular brain-derived neurotrophic factor (BDNF), which is implicated in the survival of striatal neurons. BDNF expression is reduced in Huntington's disease (HD) contributing to striatal neurodegeneration.

Initially, preclinical studies mainly discussed the neuroprotective function of MSC. Since these cells express BDNF, which is implicated in the survival of striatal neurons, its expression is reduced in Huntington's disease (HD) contributing to striatal neurodegeneration. The regenerative approaches of MSC potentially can cause the (i) promotion of endogenous neuronal growth; (ii) amelioration of the synaptic connection from damaged neurons; (iii) decrease of apoptosis of endogenous neurons; (iv) reduction of the levels of free radicals; (v) immunomodulation. Our group widely discussed these MSC functions in animal models in previous publications (**Figure 1**) [43, 44].

Furthermore, MSC can transfer larger molecules and even organelles, therefore, their use as delivery vehicles for therapeutic RNA inhibition was suggested [45]. MSC can transfer larger molecules and even organelles; therefore, suggesting their use as delivery vehicles for therapeutic RNA inhibition [45]. *In vitro* model systems showed that MSC can transfer RNAi targeting both reporter genes and mutant huntingtin in neural cell lines. Thus, the flow cytometry assay demonstrated that MSC expressing shRNA antisense to GFP decreases expression of GFP when co-cultured with SH-SY5Y cells. Furthermore, these cells, which express shRNA antisense to HTT, decreased the levels of mutant HTT expressed in both U87 and SH-SY5Y target cells

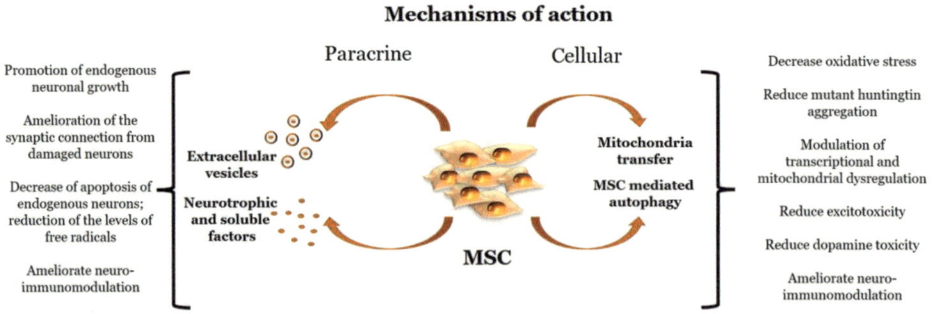

Figure 1.
Schematic representation of the paracrine and cellular mechanism of MSC action observed in pre-clinical studies in Huntington and other degenerative diseases. Paracrine action mainly includes neurotrophins and other soluble factors, including growth factors, small molecules, and cytokines, providing signals to cells and resulting in different cell actions such as survival, proliferation, and differentiation. The paracrine factors are secreted directly into the intercellular matrix or included in extracellular vesicles (exosomes) before secretion. The cellular effect includes mitochondria transfer and MSC mediated autophagy. MSC acting by paracrine and cellular mechanisms showed significant therapeutic potential.

as analyzed by Western blot and densitometry. These results are encouraging for expanding the therapeutic abilities of both RNAi and MSC for future treatments of Huntington's disease [46–48].

In addition, more recent findings suggest the potential therapeutic effect of MSC on different pathophysiological aspects of HD, such as (i) mitochondrial dysfunction; (ii) transcriptional dysregulation [49, 50]; (iii) altered axonal transport of critical factors [51, 52]; (iv) disrupted calcium signaling [53, 54]; (v) abnormal protein interactions [55]; (vi) impaired autophagy [56, 57]. However, here we will focus our review on HD mitochondrial dysfunction and MSC mitochondria transfer.

Figure 1 combines the well-known paracrine mechanism of MSC action and a novel cellular mechanism mediated by mitochondria transfer and autophagy. Both, paracrine and cellular, mechanisms provide clinical, cellular and molecular benefits in HD [43, 44, 49–59]. The complex mechanisms of MSC action and her multi-target orientation are the unique biological tool that could act on multiple pathophysiological aspects of HD cited above.

4.2.1 MSC and mitochondrial dysfunction in HD

Mitochondria roles in neurons differ from only a cell power source. Mitochondria are also dynamic organelles that fragment and fuse to achieve a maximal bioenergetics action. They are transported along microtubules, regulated intracellular calcium homeostasis through the interaction with the endoplasmic reticulum. In addition, they produce free radicals and participate in cell apoptosis [60]. These activities have been demonstrated to be changed in HD, potentially contributing to neuronal dysfunction in early pre-symptomatic HD phases. Thus, a polyglutamine-expansion disorder that primarily affects the striatum and the cerebral cortex has been described as mitochondrial dysfunction, an early pathological mechanism presenting selective HD neurodegeneration [61, 62]. One of the hallmarks of HD is an altered mitochondrial morphology that can be seen in different cell types and neurons, which are characterized by increased mitochondrial fragmentation [63]. The cells with altered mitochondrial morphology in HD cells showed a decrease in electron transport chain activity, oxygen consumption, Ca^{2+} buffering, and decreased ATP and NAD^{+} production [64]. It has been suggested that mitochondrial abnormalities can significantly affect MSNs due to the high-energy demand of this neuronal subtype [65]. Therefore, the mitochondria are a central regulatory organelle in HD-affected neurons.

In addition, mitochondria act as a reservoir for pro-apoptotic factors, thus regulating cell death. The mitochondrial permeability transition pore (mPTP) is opened due to mitochondrial dysfunction, Ca^{2+} overload, and accumulation of reactive oxygen species (ROS). The transition pore opening initiates the intrinsic apoptotic pathway, which is connected with the mitochondrial outer membrane permeabilization, awakening cytochrome c release, and activation of caspase-3 [66, 67]. Bcl-2 inhibits the activation of proapoptotic factors such as Bcl-2-associated X protein (Bax) and Bcl-2-associated K protein (Bak), thus suppressing the release of cytochrome c from mitochondria. The Bax/Bcl-2 ratio imbalance often occurs during the process of apoptosis [68]. MSC mitochondrial transfer through regulation of the balance of Bax/Bcl-2 and reduction of the expression of caspase-3 can reduce apoptosis levels and promote cell viability in recipient cells [69, 70].

Recent studies have demonstrated that MSCs have the potential to transfer the defective mitochondria between MSCs and aging cells [71]. For the first time, the MSC mitochondria transfer was shown in A549 cells with mtDNA deletions after their co-culture with human MSCs. This work demonstrated the recovery of function by mitochondrial activities such as increased oxygen consumption, membrane potential, and intracellular ATP levels [72].

It is worth mentioning that the transfer of dysfunctional mitochondria from damaged cells to MSC also can occur. Gozzelino et al. showed that mitochondria released from damaged cardiomyocytes or endothelial cells could be "swallowed" by MSCs. This event rigger increases the expression of Heme oxygenase-1 (HO-1), a protein that protects against programmed cell death, and increases mitochondria in MSCs, which in turn induces an adaptive reparative response [73, 74].

Fluorescence microscopy studies revealed MSC mitochondria transfer in astrocytes and neuron-like pheochromocytoma cells. MSC mitochondria transfer to astrocytes was more efficient when the astrocytes were subjected to ischemic damage associated with elevated ROS levels. Thc ROS accumulation in normal aging or disease leads to increasing the rate of mitophagy and decreasing the level of mitochondrial biogenesis, which reduces mitochondrial mass [75]. Such mitochondria transport re-established the bioenergetics of the recipient cells and stimulated their proliferation. Furthermore, the authors showed that MSCs mitochondria transferability may be enhanced by upregulation of Miro1 (adaptor protein participating in mitochondria moving along microtubules [76] therefore, this study showed that mitochondrial impairment in differentiated cells can be restored after MSC healthy mitochondria transfer and this approach may serve as a promising treatment for neurological diseases [77].

4.2.2 MSC mitochondria transfer and inflammation

Tissue injury or degeneration is usually followed by inflammation, which is a driving force for mitochondrial transfer. In HD, massive neuroinflammation in the striatum and caudate nucleus are already present before patients develop any symptoms [21, 78, 79]. The therapeutic effects of MSC are mediated mainly by its secretome/exosomes since in response to a combination of molecules present in the inflamed microenvironment, these cells undergo a process activation or "licensing," acquiring an anti-inflammatory phenotype and producing large amounts of immunomodulation factors, growth factors and specific chemoattractants, being able to modulate significantly innate and adaptive immune cells [38, 80].

The MSCs secreted cytokines that immunomodulate various immune cells, such as T cells, B cells, natural killer cells, and macrophages [81]. Recent studies demonstrated that between MSCs and immune cells MSC mitochondrial transfer can occur, such influencing the functions of the immune cells. Jackson et al. showed MSC mitochondria transfer occurs in an acute respiratory distress syndrome (ARDS) model. MSC provides mitochondria to host macrophages, thus enhancing the phagocytic capacity and bioenergetics of macrophages. This MSC mitochondria transfer leads to improved clearance of pathogenic bacteria [82]. Using the same model Morrison et al. showed that MSC exosomes mediated transfer of mitochondria, which can induce monocyte-derived macrophages to differentiate to an M2 phenotype with a high phagocytic capacity [58]. In addition, MSC mitochondria transfer regulates T cell differentiation. Some authors reported that when healthy donor-derived bone marrow-derived MSC (BMMSC) is cocultured with primary Th17 effector cells, the mitochondrial transfer occurs, increasing respiration in recipient Th17 cells [59].

HD demonstrates typical cellular and molecular features of inflammation, such as cytokine expression and microglia activation. However, no immune cell infiltration from the bloodstream was observed [83, 84]. Nevertheless, HD is characterized by a chronic increase of systemic pro-inflammatory cytokine production. Microglia and astrocytes are non-neuronal cells in the brain that participate in tissue homeostasis and support neuronal function. Under pathologic conditions, these cells become 'activated.' They start to produce numerous mediators promoting inflammation. These cells change their morphology and, can divide, thus increasing cell numbers, an event named 'gliosis.' Recent studies suggest that cell-autonomous pro-inflammatory activation of microglia occurs due to the expression of mutant HTT, thus contributing to the progression of HD pathogenesis [21].

MSC's metabolic state is characterized by the balance between the intrinsic necessities of the cell and limitations imposed by extrinsic conditions. Under pathogenic conditions or inflammation, MSCs respond to reactive oxygen species (ROS), damage-associated molecular patterns (DAMPs), damaged mitochondria, and mitochondrial products, thus transferring their mitochondria to damaged cells. MSC therapies can protect the potentially damaged cells by regulating cellular metabolism in injured tissues, modulating ROS and endogenous MSCs.

Furthermore, to treat such complex diseases like Huntington's, we should develop new complex therapies acting on multiple targets. MSC, due to the wide range de therapeutic molecules they produced and the different mechanisms they used to fight the disease, these cells are a good candidate for the new class of such therapeutics.

5. Cell-free therapy: novel perspectives for the treatment of HD

For a long, it was considered that the therapeutic effects of the stem cells were associated with the replacement of dead cells [73, 74]. However, in a model of kidney injury caused by the injection of toxic doses of glycerol, it was verified that transplanted stem cells remain in the injury site for up few days and, subsequently, are not found in the tissue [73, 75, 76]. These data provide evidence that the therapeutic potential of MSCs is mediated by trophic factors naturally produced and secreted by these cells in an accessible form or into EVs [1]. However, whereas the bioactive molecules present in the extracellular medium are subjected to rapid hydrolysis and oxidative effects, the biomolecules present in EVs are more stable [73]. For this reason, the EVs (particularly exosomes) have been biotechnology explored in a novel therapeutic approach known as cell-free therapy [26, 77, 78].

Cell-free therapy possesses different advantages when compared with cell-based treatment. Among these advantages are: [1] EVs can be easily prepared, stored for a relatively long period without any toxic cry preservative such as dimethylsulphoxide (DMSO) and transported; [2] therapeutic application of exosomes have been demonstrated to be well tolerated; [3] the use of EVs instead of whole cells avoids possible complications associated with pulmonary embolism after intravenous infusion of MSCs; [4] avoids the risk of unlimited cell growth and tumor formation since EVs are not dividing; [5] exosomes from MSCs, and epithelial cells do not induce toxicity when repeatedly injected; [6] EV may be isolated from unmodified or genetically modified human stem cells; [7] evaluation of culture medium for safety and efficacy is much simpler and analogous to conventional pharmaceutical agents [1, 73, 79–82]. Further, the cell-free therapy allows biotechnologically exploring the use of the culture medium, which is generally discarded as a byproduct of the in vitro expansion of MSCs. This is because this culture medium—also termed conditioned medium (CM) [79]—is an essential source of bioactive molecules, which can find in an accessible form or an extracellular vesicle (EVs) [1].

5.1 Perspectives and challenges in cell-free therapy

Although, different strategies have been successfully used to isolate exosomes, they represent the main obstacle to the therapeutic application of EV since these procedures are time-consuming and generally provide few quantities of EVs [1, 73]. However, novel methodologies have been proposed to solve these problems. Based on this, we aimed to summarize the pros and cons of each available method for isolating exosomes.

Ultracentrifugation (UC) and commercial kit rooted in polymer-based precipitation are the most well-established and standard methods used for isolating exosomes [74], being adopted as a strategy in about 81% of researches [78]. Ultracentrifugation-based methods can be divided into two major types of techniques according to the separation mechanism: (i) differential ultracentrifugation and (ii) density gradient ultracentrifugation [78]. For both methods, death cells, cellular debris, and large EVs (>200 nm) are separated using low centrifugal forces (300–2000 × *g*) for 10–30 min at room temperature, as verified in the most protocol, as already revised by us [1]. An additional filtration step using a 0.22–0.45 μm-membrane filter can increase the exosome purity. In differential ultracentrifugation, the particles are separated using a serial of differential centrifugal forces (100,000–120,000 × *g*) and time (70 min to 12 h). At the end of the process, the pellet of exosomes is washed with phosphate saline buffer (PBS) or 0.9% NaCl solution to remove remaining proteins co-isolated with the EVs. Differential ultracentrifugation provides pure EVs for both scientific and clinical purposes. However, the majorities of UC-based proposed methods are laborious, time-consuming, and unsuitable for mass-scale EV production, making it difficult for therapeutics [1]. In density gradient, ultracentrifugation (DGUC) is employed as a sucrose density gradient, which reduces the destructive effects of centrifugal force on exosomes [58, 78]. According to the exosome buoyant density in aqueous sucrose (1.10–1.20 g/mL), the exosomes can be easily isolated [59, 78]. Although, this method provides the highest efficiency for exosome purification, its suitability for clinical purposes is questionable due to the difficulty in upscaling and automating the process [83, 84]. Moreover, the wash step is mandatory for this method to remove eventual residues of CsCl or sucrose used to obtain the gradient density.

Another strategy commonly employed to isolate exosomes is coprecipitation. This method uses polymers, such as polyethylene glycol (PEG) 6000 or 8000, which can coprecipitate with hydrophobic proteins and lipid molecules present in exosome membranes [78]. Although, most simple and less expensive than the methods based on ultracentrifugation, the isolation using coprecipitation is not scalable, limiting its use for therapeutic purposes. Moreover, this technique requires sample incubation with the polymers for a long time (generally 12–16 h) [1].

The differential expression of specific surface biomarkers, such as CD9, CD63, and CD83, also provides an excellent opportunity to develop immunoaffinity-capture-based techniques for exosomes isolation using modified magnetic beads or micro-channels surfaces with specific antibodies [1, 78]. Although, this technique allows isolating only exosomes, it works with few volumes, limiting its use for therapeutic purposes, which require scalable methods. Moreover, this method generally requires a pre-enrichment step, which is commonly performed using commercial kits based on coprecipitation, resulting in PEG contamination [1].

Another strategy used to isolate exosomes is the size-based isolation technique. This technique can be based on sequential filtration, size-exclusion chromatography (SEC), and size-dependent microfluids. These methods allow isolating the EVs according to their size [78]. EVs are separated using membrane filters with different size or molecular weight exclusion limits in sequential filtration. First, the CM is filtered using a 0.22 μm membrane filter. Then, proteins with a 500 kDa molecular weight are purified using a dialysis bag. Finally, the samples are filtered with a 100 nm membrane filter [78]. The SEC is based on particle size filtration through a porous stationary phase composed of spherical gel beads with pores of specific size [78]. Large particles are eluted when the sample passes through the stationary phase, whereas small particles pass through the pores [78]. The size-dependent microfluidics uses a viscoelastic microfluidics device, composed of a microchannel, two inlets, and three inlets, to fractionate exosomes from other types of EVs [78]. These techniques are faster than those based on ultracentrifugation and do not require special equipment. Moreover, they avoid PEG contamination, frequently observed in coprecipitation-based methods. However, the size-based isolation techniques are relatively expensive and cannot separate exosomes from other EVs, requiring additional steps for exosome purification [1].

5.2 Cell-free therapy for the treatment of HD

Due to their ability to cross the blood-brain barrier and biocompatibility, exosomes are promising therapeutic drug carriers into the CNS. In HD, exosomes are exceptionally efficient in delivering specific microRNAs (miRs), short non-coding RNAs of about 22 nucleotides that regulate gene expression by suppressing the translation of mRNA, which are found deregulated in HD patients.

In this sense, several miRs had already been identified as deregulated in HD, including the miR-124, which was found downregulated in HD patients [85]. The decreased expression of miR-124 increases the levels of its target gene (REST), which acts as a repressor of BDNF [85]. By contrast, the expression of miR-124 induces adult neurogenesis in the subventricular zone (SVZ) and regulates the cell cycle in striatal neurons. Considering that the HD striatum exhibits decreased neurogenesis, which leads to brain atrophy, it was hypothesized that the delivery of miR-124 may be a feasible way to induce neural regeneration. However, naked miRs are vulnerable to degradation.

In this regard, exosomes emerge as candidates for the miR-124 delivery to recipient cells. Based on this, Lee et al. [85] injected exosomes derived from HEK 293 cells overexpressing miR-124 within (Exo-124) the striatum of 6-week-old R6/2 transgenic mice. Using ex vivo imaging, the authors demonstrated the presence and maintenance of the exosomes within the striatum even after one week later the Exo-124 administration. Furthermore, it was verified that Exo-124-treated R6/2 mice exhibited slightly higher levels of miR-124 when compared to the non-treated mice (control). However, no statistically significant differences between the treated and control mice were reported. By contrast, the Exo-124-treated R6/2 mice exhibited lower levels of REST protein concerning the control. Although, the study had provided a proof of concept for exosome-based delivery of miRNAs to the brain, the therapeutic efficacy of Exo-124 was modest, suggesting the need to increase the dose of miRNAs packed in the exosomes or to combine this miRNA with other candidate miRNAs such as miR-9, miR-22, miR-125b, miR-146a, miR-150, and miR-214.

In this sense, the exosomes derived from MSCs can be considered an important source of these miRs and other mRNAs and proteins deregulated in HD physiopathology. Supporting this, Lee et al. [86] showed that exosomes derived from an adipose-derived stem cell (ASC-exo) decreased mHtt aggregates in R6/2 mice-derived neuronal cells through the upregulation of PGC-1, phospho-CREB.

6. Conclusion

In this review, we demonstrated that Huntington's disease is devastating and affects brain cells and the organism as a whole. Although, the main cause of HD patients' death is medium spiny neurons, many specific events occur at presymptomatic and symptomatic HD phases. Currently, Huntington's chorea is in the focus of pharmaceutical companies, producing drugs able to combat this HD symptom. However, these drugs are always not possible to delay the disease and present moderate to severe side effects.

In contrast to conventional drugs, MSC is safe, and they did not present any side effects as shown in multiple clinical trials. MSC showed therapeutic potential distinct from, for example, small molecules and biologics. Cells are deposited multiple drugs, they can sense diverse signals, migrate to specific sites in the body, make decisions, and carry out complex responses inside one specific tissue environment.

Our knowledge about the biology and therapeutic potential of these cells is still minimal; however, as demonstrated by scientific literature, these cells and their derivatives as exosomes and mitochondria have tremendous therapeutic potential. Pre-clinical studies provided evidence about the paracrine effect of these cells' such as regenerative, anti-apoptotic, anti-fibrotic anti-inflammatory, immunosuppressive, immunomodulatory, and angiogenic.

More recently, the potential effect of MSC against different pathophysiological aspects of HD, such as mitochondrial dysfunction; transcriptional dysregulation; altered axonal transport of critical factors; disrupted calcium signaling; abnormal protein interactions, and impaired autophagy, has been demonstrated.

This review tries to provide insight into cellular and cell-free technologies from the exact cellular origin. These cell and cell-free products may share similar features and present specific characteristics, as demonstrated for MSC, exosomes, and mitochondria. We tried to clarify that these products aim at different cellular targets or molecular pathways involved in Huntington's disease. Therefore, we should study how to use these new therapeutics, which can delay or even stop neurodegenerative devasting diseases.

Author details

Irina Kerkis[1]*, Rodrigo Pinheiro Araldi[2], Cristiane Valverde Wenceslau[3] and Thais Biude Mendes[1]

1 Genetics Laboratory, Butantan Institute, São Paulo, Brazil

2 Federal University of São Paulo, Cellavita Pesquisas Científicas, São Paulo, Brazil

3 Cellavita Pesquisas Científicas, Valinhos, SP, Brazil

*Address all correspondence to: irina.kerkis@butantan.gov.br

References

[1] Araldi RP, D'Amelio F, Vigerelli H, de Melo TC, Kerkis I. Stem cell-derived exosomes as therapeutic approach for neurodegenerative Ddsorders: From biology to biotechnology. Cell. 2020;**9**(12):2663. Available from: https://www.mdpi.com/2073-4409/9/12/2663

[2] Lee J-M, Correia K, Loupe J, Kim K-H, Barker D, Hong EP, et al. CAG repeat not polyglutamine length determines timing of Huntington's disease onset. Cell. 2019;**178**(4):887-900.e14. Available from: https://linkinghub.elsevier.com/retrieve/pii/S0092867419307391

[3] Jimenez-Sanchez M, Licitra F, Underwood BR, Rubinsztein DC. Huntington's disease: Mechanisms of pathogenesis and therapeutic strategies. Cold Spring Harbor Perspectives in Medicine. 2017;**7**(7):a024240. Available from: http://perspectivesinmedicine.cshlp.org/lookup/doi/10.1101/cshperspect.a024240

[4] Langbehn DR, Hayden MR, Paulsen JS. CAG-repeat length and the age of onset in Huntington disease (HD): A review and validation study of statistical approaches. American Journal of Medical Genetics. Part B, Neuropsychiatric Genetics. 2010;**153B**(2):397-408. Available from: http://doi.wiley.com/10.1002/ajmg.b.30992

[5] Schulte J, Littleton JT. The biological function of the huntingtin protein and its relevance to Huntington's disease pathology. Current Trends in Neurology. 2011;**5**:65-78. Available from: https://pubmed.ncbi.nlm.nih.gov/22180703

[6] Shimojo M. Huntingtin regulates RE1-silencing transcription factor/neuron-restrictive silencer factor (REST/NRSF) nuclear trafficking indirectly through a complex with REST/NRSF-interacting LIM domain protein (RILP) and dynactin p150Glued. The Journal of Biological Chemistry. 2008;**283**(50):34880-34886. Available from: https://linkinghub.elsevier.com/retrieve/pii/S0021925820633117

[7] Ravache M, Weber C, Mérienne K, Trottier Y. Transcriptional activation of REST by Sp1 in Huntington's disease models. Feany MB, editor. PLoS One. 2010;**5**(12):e14311. Available from: https://dx.plos.org/10.1371/journal.pone.0014311

[8] Oliveira JMA, Jekabsons MB, Chen S, Lin A, Rego AC, Gonçalves J, et al. Mitochondrial dysfunction in Huntington's disease: The bioenergetics of isolated and in situ mitochondria from transgenic mice. Journal of Neurochemistry. 2007;**101**(1):241-249. Available from: https://onlinelibrary.wiley.com/doi/10.1111/j.1471-4159.2006.04361.x

[9] Hunt RJ, Bateman JM. Mitochondrial retrograde signaling in the nervous system. FEBS Letters. 2018;**592**(5):663-678. Available from: https://onlinelibrary.wiley.com/doi/10.1002/1873-3468.12890

[10] Quintanilla RA, Johnson GVW. Role of mitochondrial dysfunction in the pathogenesis of Huntington's disease. Brain Research Bulletin. 2009;**80**(4-5):242-247. Available from: https://linkinghub.elsevier.com/retrieve/pii/S0361923009002184

[11] Carmo C, Naia L, Lopes C, Rego AC. Mitochondrial dysfunction in Huntington's disease. Advances in Experimental Medicine and Biology. 2018;**1049**:59-83. Available from: http://link.springer.com/10.1007/978-3-319-71779-1_3

[12] Chaturvedi RK, Hennessey T, Johri A, Tiwari SK, Mishra D, Agarwal S, et al. Transducer of regulated CREB-binding proteins (TORCs) transcription and function is impaired in Huntington's disease. Human Molecular Genetics. 2012;**21**(15):3474-3488. Available from: https://academic.oup.com/hmg/article-lookup/doi/10.1093/hmg/dds178

[13] Jeong H, Cohen DE, Cui L, Supinski A, Savas JN, Mazzulli JR, et al. Sirt1 mediates neuroprotection from mutant huntingtin by activation of the TORC1 and CREB transcriptional pathway. Nature Medicine. 2012;**18**(1):159-165. Available from: http://www.nature.com/articles/nm.2559

[14] Johri A, Chandra A, Flint BM. PGC-1α, mitochondrial dysfunction, and Huntington's disease. Free Radical Biology & Medicine. 2013;**62**:37-46. Available from: https://linkinghub.elsevier.com/retrieve/pii/S0891584913001561

[15] Bossy-Wetzel E, Petrilli A, Knott AB. Mutant huntingtin and mitochondrial dysfunction. Trends in Neurosciences. 2008;**31**(12):609-616. Available from: https://linkinghub.elsevier.com/retrieve/pii/S0166223608002129

[16] Hsiao H-Y, Chen Y-C, Chen H-M, Tu P-H, Chern Y. A critical role of astrocyte-mediated nuclear factor-κB-dependent inflammation in Huntington's disease. Human Molecular Genetics. 2013;**22**(9):1826-1842. Available from: https://academic.oup.com/hmg/article-lookup/doi/10.1093/hmg/ddt036

[17] Marcora E, Kennedy MB. The Huntington's disease mutation impairs Huntingtin's role in the transport of NF-κB from the synapse to the nucleus. Human Molecular Genetics. 2010;**19**(22):4373-4384. Available from: https://academic.oup.com/hmg/article-lookup/doi/10.1093/hmg/ddq358

[18] Wu S-Y, Pan B-S, Tsai S-F, Chiang Y-T, Huang B-M, Mo F-E, et al. BDNF reverses aging-related microglial activation. Journal of Neuroinflammation. 2020;**17**(1):210. Available from: https://jneuroinflammation.biomedcentral.com/articles/10.1186/s12974-020-01887-1

[19] Palpagama TH, Waldvogel HJ, Faull RLM, Kwakowsky A. The role of microglia and astrocytes in Huntington's disease. Frontiers in Molecular Neuroscience. 2019;**12**:258. Available from: https://www.frontiersin.org/article/10.3389/fnmol.2019.00258/full

[20] Lois C, González I, Izquierdo-García D, Zürcher NR, Wilkens P, Loggia ML, et al. Neuroinflammation in Huntington's disease: New insights with 11 C-PBR28 PET/MRI. ACS Chemical Neuroscience. 2018;**9**(11):2563-2571. Available from: https://pubs.acs.org/doi/10.1021/acschemneuro.8b00072

[21] Crotti A, Glass CK. The choreography of neuroinflammation in Huntington's disease. Trends in Immunology. 2015;**36**(6):364-373. Available from: https://linkinghub.elsevier.com/retrieve/pii/S1471490615001040

[22] Hunter M, Demarais NJ, Faull RLM, Grey AC, Curtis MA. Subventricular zone lipidomic architecture loss in Huntington's disease. Journal of Neurochemistry. 2018;**146**(5):613-630. Available from: https://onlinelibrary.wiley.com/doi/10.1111/jnc.14468

[23] Kandasamy M, Rosskopf M, Wagner K, Klein B, Couillard-Despres S, Reitsamer HA, et al. Reduction in subventricular zone-derived olfactory bulb neurogenesis in a rat model of Huntington's disease is accompanied by striatal invasion of neuroblasts. Szele F, editor. PLoS One. 2015;**10**(2):e0116069. Available from: https://dx.plos.org/10.1371/journal.pone.0116069

[24] Kandasamy M, Aigner L. Reactive Neuroblastosis in Huntington's disease: A putative therapeutic target for striatal regeneration in the adult brain. Frontiers in Cellular Neuroscience. 2018;**12**:37. Available from: http://journal.frontiersin.org/article/10.3389/fncel.2018.00037/full

[25] da Costa VR, Araldi RP, Vigerelli H, D'Ámelio F, Mendes TB, Gonzaga V, et al. Exosomes in the tumor microenvironment: From biology to clinical applications. Cell. 2021;**10**(10):2617. Available from: https://www.mdpi.com/2073-4409/10/10/2617

[26] Gomez-Salazar M, Gonzalez-Galofre ZN, Casamitjana J, Crisan M, James AW, Péault B. Five decades later, are mesenchymal stem cells still relevant? Frontiers in Bioengineering and Biotechnology. 2020;**8**:148. Available from: https://www.frontiersin.org/article/10.3389/fbioe.2020.00148/full

[27] Bianco P, Robey O, Simmons P. Mesenchymal stem cells: Revisiting history, concepts and assays. Cell Stem Cell. 2008;**2**(4):313-319

[28] Robinton DA, Daley GQ. The promise of induced pluripotent stem cells in research and therapy. Nature. 2012;**481**(7381):295-305. Available from: http://www.nature.com/articles/nature10761

[29] Pittenger MF, Discher DE, Péault BM, Phinney DG, Hare JM, Caplan AI. Mesenchymal stem cell perspective: Cell biology to clinical progress. Npj. Regenerative Medicine. 2019;**4**(1):22. Available from: http://www.nature.com/articles/s41536-019-0083-6

[30] Caplan AI. MSCs: The sentinel and safe-guards of injury. Journal of Cellular Physiology. 2016;**231**(7):1413-1416. Available from: https://onlinelibrary.wiley.com/doi/10.1002/jcp.25255

[31] Caplan AI, Sorrell JM. The MSC curtain that stops the immune system. Immunology Letters. 2015;**168**(2):136-139. Available from: https://linkinghub.elsevier.com/retrieve/pii/S0165247815001030

[32] Weiss ARR, Dahlke MH. Immunomodulation by mesenchymal stem cells (MSCs): Mechanisms of action of living, apoptotic, and dead MSCs. Frontiers in Immunology. 2019;**10**:1-10. Available from: https://www.frontiersin.org/article/10.3389/fimmu.2019.01191/full

[33] Kassis I, Grigoriadis N, Gowda-Kurkalli B, Mizrachi-Kol R, Ben-Hur T, Slavin S, et al. Neuroprotection and immunomodulation with mesenchymal stem cells in chronic experimental autoimmune encephalomyelitis. Archives of Neurology. 2008;**65**(6):753-761. Available from: http://archneur.jamanetwork.com/article.aspx?doi=10.1001/archneur.65.6.753

[34] Yu-Taeger L, Stricker-Shaver J, Arnold K, Bambynek-Dziuk P, Novati A, Singer E, et al. Intranasal administration of mesenchymal stem cells ameliorates the abnormal dopamine transmission system and inflammatory reaction in the R6/2 mouse model of Huntington disease. Cell. 2019;**8**(6):595. Available from: https://www.mdpi.com/2073-4409/8/6/595

[35] Gothelf Y, Kaspi H, Abramov N, Aricha R. miRNA profiling of NurOwn®: Mesenchymal stem cells secreting neurotrophic factors. Stem Cell Research & Therapy. 2017;**8**(1):249. Available from: https://stemcellres.biomedcentral.com/articles/10.1186/s13287-017-0692-1

[36] Kim YR, Ahn SM, Pak ME, Lee HJ, Jung DH, Shin Y-I, et al. Potential benefits of mesenchymal stem cells and electroacupuncture on the trophic factors associated with neurogenesis in mice with ischemic stroke. Scientific Reports. 2018;**8**(1):2044. Available from: http://www.nature.com/articles/s41598-018-20481-3

[37] Caplan AI. Mesenchymal stem cells: Time to change the name! Stem Cells Translational Medicine. 2017;**6**(6):1445-1451. Available from: https://academic.oup.com/stcltm/article/6/6/1445/6448531

[38] Le Blanc K, Mougiakakos D. Multipotent mesenchymal stromal cells and the innate immune system. Nature Reviews. Immunology. 2012;**12**(5):383-396. Available from: http://www.nature.com/articles/nri3209

[39] Parekkadan B, Milwid JM. Mesenchymal stem cells as therapeutics. Annual Review of Biomedical Engineering. 2010;**12**(1):87-117. Available from: http://www.annualreviews.org/doi/10.1146/annurev-bioeng-070909-105309

[40] Bernardo ME, Fibbe WE. Mesenchymal stromal cells: Sensors and switchers of inflammation. Cell Stem Cell. 2013;**13**(4):392-402. Available from: https://linkinghub.elsevier.com/retrieve/pii/S1934590913004062

[41] Dominici M, Le Blanc K, Mueller I, Slaper-Cortenbach I, Marini F, Krause D, et al. Minimal criteria for defining multipotent mesenchymal stromal cells. The International Society for Cellular Therapy position statement. Cytotherapy. 2006;**8**(4):315-317. Available from: https://www.tandfonline.com/doi/abs/10.1080/14653240600855905

[42] Le Blanc K, Davies LC. MSCs—Cells with many sides. Cytotherapy. 2018;**20**(3):273-278. Available from: https://linkinghub.elsevier.com/retrieve/pii/S146532491830015X

[43] Kerkis I, Macedo da Silva J, Valverde Wenceslau C, Caroline Mambelli-Lisboa N, Osorio FE. Brain-derived neurotrophic factor and stem cell-based technologies in Huntington's disease therapy. In: Neurodegenerative Diseases—Molecular Mechanisms and Current Therapeutic Approaches [Working Title]. London, UK: IntechOpen; 2020

[44] Kerkis I, Haddad MS, Valverde CW, Glosman S. Neural and mesenchymal stem cells in animal models of Huntington's disease: Past experiences and future challenges. Stem Cell Research & Therapy. 2015;**6**(1):232. Available from: https://stemcellres.biomedcentral.com/articles/10.1186/s13287-015-0248-1

[45] Meyerrose TE, Roberts M, Ohlemiller KK, Vogler CA, Wirthlin L, Nolta JA, et al. Lentiviral-transduced human mesenchymal stem cells persistently express therapeutic levels of enzyme in a xenotransplantation model of human disease. Stem Cells. 2008;**26**(7):1713-1722. Available from: https://onlinelibrary.wiley.com/doi/10.1634/stemcells.2008-0008

[46] Esmaeilzadeh A, Farshbaf A. Mesenchymal stem cell as a vector for gene and cell therapy strategies. Studies on Stem Cells Research and Therapy. 2015;**1**(1):017-018. Available from: https://www.peertechz.com/articles/SSCRT-1-105.php

[47] Meyerrose T, Olson S, Pontow S, Kalomoiris S, Jung Y, Annett G, et al. Mesenchymal stem cells for the sustained in vivo delivery of bioactive factors. Advanced Drug Delivery Reviews.

2010;**62**(12):1167-1174. Available from: https://linkinghub.elsevier.com/retrieve/pii/S0169409X10001912

[48] Joyce N, Annett G, Wirthlin L, Olson S, Bauer G, Nolta JA. Mesenchymal stem cells for the treatment of neurodegenerative disease. Regenerative Medicine. 2010;**5**(6):933-946. Available from: https://www.futuremedicine.com/doi/10.2217/rme.10.72

[49] Kumar A, Vaish M, Ratan RR. Transcriptional dysregulation in Huntington's disease: A failure of adaptive transcriptional homeostasis. Drug Discovery Today. 2014;**19**(7):956-962. Available from: https://linkinghub.elsevier.com/retrieve/pii/S1359644614000932

[50] Im W, Ban J, Lim J, Lee M, Lee S-T, Chu K, et al. Extracts of adipose derived stem cells slows progression in the R6/2 model of Huntington's disease. Reddy H, editor. PLoS One. 2013;**8**(4):e59438. Available from: https://dx.plos.org/10.1371/journal.pone.0059438

[51] Chevalier-Larsen E, Holzbaur ELF. Axonal transport and neurodegenerative disease. Biochimica et Biophysica Acta (BBA)—Molecular Basis of Disease. 2006;**1762**(11-12):1094-1108. Available from: https://linkinghub.elsevier.com/retrieve/pii/S0925443906000731

[52] Oh SH, Lee SC, Kim DY, Kim HN, Shin JY, Ye BS, et al. Mesenchymal stem cells stabilize axonal transports for Autophagic clearance of α-Synuclein in parkinsonian models. Stem Cells. 2017;**35**(8):1934-1947. Available from: https://academic.oup.com/stmcls/article/35/8/1934/6453251

[53] Elbaz EM, Helmy HS, El-Sahar AE, Saad MA, Sayed RH. Lercanidipine boosts the efficacy of mesenchymal stem cell therapy in 3-NP-induced Huntington's disease model rats via modulation of the calcium/calcineurin/NFATc4 and Wnt/β-catenin signalling pathways. Neurochemistry International. 2019;**131**:104548. Available from: https://linkinghub.elsevier.com/retrieve/pii/S0197018619303377

[54] Czeredys M. Dysregulation of neuronal calcium signaling via store-operated channels in Huntington's disease. Front cell Developmental Biology. 2020;**8**:11735. Available from: https://www.frontiersin.org/articles/10.3389/fcell.2020.611735/full

[55] Wanker EE, Ast A, Schindler F, Trepte P, Schnoegl S. The pathobiology of perturbed mutant huntingtin protein–protein interactions in Huntington's disease. Journal of Neurochemistry. 2019;**151**(4):507-519. Available from: https://onlinelibrary.wiley.com/doi/10.1111/jnc.14853

[56] Croce KR, Yamamoto A. A role for autophagy in Huntington's disease. Neurobiology of Disease. 2019;**122**:16-22. Available from: https://linkinghub.elsevier.com/retrieve/pii/S0969996118304819

[57] Ceccariglia S, Cargnoni A, Silini AR, Parolini O. Autophagy: A potential key contributor to the therapeutic action of mesenchymal stem cells. Autophagy. 2020;**16**(1):28-37. Available from: https://linkinghub.elsevier.com/retrieve/pii/S0969996118304819

[58] Morrison TJ, Jackson MV, Cunningham EK, Kissenpfennig A, McAuley DF, O'Kane CM, et al. Mesenchymal stromal cells modulate macrophages in clinically relevant lung injury models by extracellular vesicle mitochondrial transfer. American Journal of Respiratory and Critical Care Medicine. 2017;**196**(10):1275-1286. Available from: http://www.atsjournals.org/doi/10.1164/rccm.201701-0170OC

[59] Luz-Crawford P, Hernandez J, Djouad F, Luque-Campos N, Caicedo A, Carrère-Kremer S, et al. Mesenchymal stem cell repression of Th17 cells is triggered by mitochondrial transfer. Stem Cell Research & Therapy. 2019;**10**(1):232. Available from: https://stemcellres.biomedcentral.com/articles/10.1186/s13287-019-1307-9

[60] Bhatti JS, Bhatti GK, Reddy PH. Mitochondrial dysfunction and oxidative stress in metabolic disorders—A step towards mitochondria based therapeutic strategies. Biochimica et Biophysica Acta (BBA)—Molecular Basis of Disease. 2017;**1863**(5):1066-1077. Available from: https://linkinghub.elsevier.com/retrieve/pii/S0925443916302927

[61] Dubinsky JM. Towards an understanding of energy impairment in Huntington's disease brain. Journal of Huntington's Disease. 2017;**6**(4):267-302. Available from: https://www.medra.org/servlet/aliasResolver?alias=iospress&doi=10.3233/JHD-170264

[62] Costa V, Scorrano L. Shaping the role of mitochondria in the pathogenesis of Huntington's disease. The EMBO Journal. 2012;**31**(8):1853-1864. Available from: http://emboj.embopress.org/cgi/doi/10.1038/emboj.2012.65

[63] Kim J, Moody JP, Edgerly CK, Bordiuk OL, Cormier K, Smith K, et al. Mitochondrial loss, dysfunction and altered dynamics in Huntington's disease. Human Molecular Genetics. 2010;**19**(20):3919-3935. Available from: https://academic.oup.com/hmg/article-lookup/doi/10.1093/hmg/ddq306

[64] Oliveira JMA. Nature and cause of mitochondrial dysfunction in Huntington's disease: Focusing on huntingtin and the striatum. Journal of Neurochemistry. 2010;**114**:1-12. Available from: https://onlinelibrary.wiley.com/doi/10.1111/j.1471-4159.2010.06741.x

[65] Pickrell AM, Fukui H, Wang X, Pinto M, Moraes CT. The striatum is highly susceptible to mitochondrial oxidative phosphorylation dysfunctions. The Journal of Neuroscience. 2011;**31**(27):9895-9904. Available from: https://www.jneurosci.org/lookup/doi/10.1523/JNEUROSCI.6223-10.2011

[66] Dumollard R, Carroll J, Duchen MR, Campbell K, Swann K. Mitochondrial function and redox state in mammalian embryos. Seminars in Cell & Developmental Biology. 2009;**20**(3):346-353. Available from: https://linkinghub.elsevier.com/retrieve/pii/S1084952109000032

[67] Quintanilla RA, Tapia C, Pérez MJ. Possible role of mitochondrial permeability transition pore in the pathogenesis of Huntington disease. Biochemical and Biophysical Research Communications. 2017;**483**(4):1078-1083. Available from: https://linkinghub.elsevier.com/retrieve/pii/S0006291X16315145

[68] Xie L, Wu Y, Fan Z, Liu Y, Zeng J. Astragalus polysaccharide protects human cardiac microvascular endothelial cells from hypoxia/reoxygenation injury: The role of PI3K/AKT, Bax/Bcl-2 and caspase-3. Molecular Medicine Reports. 2016;**14**(1):904-910. Available from: https://www.spandidos-publications.com/10.3892/mmr.2016.5296

[69] Konari N, Nagaishi K, Kikuchi S, Fujimiya M. Mitochondria transfer from mesenchymal stem cells structurally and functionally repairs renal proximal tubular epithelial cells in diabetic nephropathy in vivo. Scientific Reports. 2019;**9**(1):5184. Available

from: http://www.nature.com/articles/s41598-019-40163-y

[70] Han H, Hu J, Yan Q, Zhu J, Zhu Z, Chen Y, et al. Bone marrow-derived mesenchymal stem cells rescue injured H9c2 cells via transferring intact mitochondria through tunneling nanotubes in an in vitro simulated ischemia/reperfusion model. Molecular Medicine Reports. 2016;**13**(2):1517-1524. Available from: https://www.spandidos-publications.com/10.3892/mmr.2015.4726

[71] Li C, Cheung MKH, Han S, Zhang Z, Chen L, Chen J, et al. Mesenchymal stem cells and their mitochondrial transfer: A double-edged sword. Bioscience Reports. 2019;**39**(5):BSR20182417. Available from: https://portlandpress.com/bioscirep/article/39/5/BSR20182417/219196/Mesenchymal-stem-cells-and-their-mitochondrial

[72] Spees JL, Olson SD, Whitney MJ, Prockop DJ. Mitochondrial transfer between cells can rescue aerobic respiration. Proceedings of the National Academy of Sciences. 2006;**103**(5):1283-1288. Available from: http://www.pnas.org/cgi/doi/10.1073/pnas.0510511103

[73] Gozzelino R, Jeney V, Soares MP. Mechanisms of cell protection by Heme Oxygenase-1. Annual Review of Pharmacology and Toxicology. 2010;**50**(1):323-354. Available from: https://www.annualreviews.org/doi/10.1146/annurev.pharmtox.010909.105600

[74] Mahrouf-Yorgov M, Augeul L, Da Silva CC, Jourdan M, Rigolet M, Manin S, et al. Mesenchymal stem cells sense mitochondria released from damaged cells as danger signals to activate their rescue properties. Cell Death and Differentiation. 2017;**24**(7):1224-1238. Available from: http://www.nature.com/articles/cdd201751

[75] Angelova PR, Barilani M, Lovejoy C, Dossena M, Viganò M, Seresini A, et al. Mitochondrial dysfunction in parkinsonian mesenchymal stem cells impairs differentiation. Redox Biology. 2018;**14**:474-484. Available from: https://linkinghub.elsevier.com/retrieve/pii/S2213231717307437

[76] Babenko V, Silachev D, Popkov V, Zorova L, Pevzner I, Plotnikov E, et al. Miro1 enhances mitochondria transfer from multipotent mesenchymal stem cells (MMSC) to neural cells and improves the efficacy of cell recovery. Molecules. 2018;**23**(3):687. Available from: http://www.mdpi.com/1420-3049/23/3/687

[77] Han D, Zheng X, Wang X, Jin T, Cui L, Chen Z. Mesenchymal stem/stromal cell-mediated mitochondrial transfer and the therapeutic potential in treatment of neurological diseases. Stem Cells International. 2020;**2020**:1-16. Available from: https://www.hindawi.com/journals/sci/2020/8838046/

[78] Agus F, Crespo D, Myers RH, Labadorf A. The caudate nucleus undergoes dramatic and unique transcriptional changes in human prodromal Huntington's disease brain. BMC Medical Genomics. 2019;**12**(137):1-17

[79] Soulet D, Cicchetti F. The role of immunity in Huntington's disease. Molecular Psychiatry. 2011;**16**(9):889-902. Available from: http://www.nature.com/articles/mp201128

[80] Qi K, Li N, Zhang Z, Melino G. Tissue regeneration: The crosstalk between mesenchymal stem cells and immune response. Cellular Immunology. 2018;**326**:86-93. Available from: https://linkinghub.elsevier.com/retrieve/pii/S0008874917302198

[81] Kovach TK, Dighe AS, Lobo PI, Cui Q. Interactions between MSCs and immune cells: Implications for bone healing. Journal of Immunology Research. 2015;**2015**:1-17. Available from: http://www.hindawi.com/journals/jir/2015/752510/

[82] Jackson MV, Morrison TJ, Doherty DF, McAuley DF, Matthay MA, Kissenpfennig A, et al. Mitochondrial transfer via tunneling nanotubes is an important mechanism by which mesenchymal stem cells enhance macrophage phagocytosis in the in vitro and in vivo models of ARDS. Stem Cells. 2016;**34**(8):2210-2223. Available from: https://onlinelibrary.wiley.com/doi/10.1002/stem.2372

[83] Silvestroni A, Faull RLM, Strand AD, Möller T. Distinct neuroinflammatory profile in post-mortem human Huntington's disease. Neuroreport. 2009;**20**(12):1098-1103. Available from: https://journals.lww.com/00001756-200908050-00012

[84] Andre R, Carty L, Tabrizi SJ. Disruption of immune cell function by mutant huntingtin in Huntington's disease pathogenesis. Current Opinion in Pharmacology. 2016;**26**:33-38. Available from: https://linkinghub.elsevier.com/retrieve/pii/S1471489215001101

[85] Lee S-T, Im W, Ban J-J, Lee M, Jung K-H, Lee SK, et al. Exosome-based delivery of miR-124 in a Huntington's disease model. Journal of Movement Disorders [Internet]. 2017 Jan 25;**10**(1):45-52. Available from: http://e-jmd.org/journal/view.php?doi=10.14802/jmd.16054

[86] Lee M, Liu T, Im W, Kim M. In Smith Y, editor. Exosomes from adipose-derived stem cells ameliorate phenotype of Huntington's disease in vitro model. European Journal of Neuroscience [Internet]. 2016;**44**(4):2114-2119. Available from: https://onlinelibrary.wiley.com/doi/10.1111/ejn.13275

Chapter 7

Nrf2 as a Potential Therapeutic Target for Treatment of Huntington's Disease

Saravanan Jayaram, Praveen Thaggikuppe Krishnamurthy, Meghana Joshi and Vishnu Kumar

Abstract

Oxidative stress-induced neuronal damage plays a significant role in pathogenesis of several neuro-degenerative disorders including Huntington's disease. In Huntington's disease, oxidative stress-induced neuronal damage is reported to be mediated by PGC-1α and microglial cells. This development led to various clinical trials that tested the efficacy of several exogenous antioxidants such as vitamin E, vitamin C, etc. to prevent the oxidative stress-induced cell damage in several neuro-degenerative disorders. But these randomized clinical trials did not find any significant beneficial effects of exogenous antioxidants in neuro-degenerative disorders. This forced scientists to search endogenous targets that would enhance the production of antioxidants. Nrf2 is one such ideal target that increases the transcription of genes involved in production of antioxidants. Nrf2 is a transcription factor that controls the expression of antioxidant genes that defend cells against oxidative stress. This chapter focuses on the role of oxidative stress in Huntington's disease and explores the therapeutic benefits of Nrf2 activators.

Keywords: Nrf2, oxidative stress, Keap 1, Huntington's disease

1. Introduction

Huntington's disease is an inherited autosomal dominant neurodegenerative disorder characterized by a triad of psychiatric, cognitive and motor symptoms. Every human has two copies of the huntingtin gene (HTT) that codes for huntingtin protein (htt) [1]. The exact functions of huntingtin protein still remain unclear, but it is believed to be involved in the development and formation of cortical and striatal excitatory synapses, surveillance and biogenesis of mitochondrial function, activation of glial cells, upregulation of the expression of brain derived neurotrophic factor, balance of histone acetylation and deacetylation, axonal transport, regulation of signaling pathways and autophagy [2–5]. The HTT gene, also called as *IT15* ('interesting transcript 15') gene, is located on the short arm (p) of chromosome number 4 at 4p16.3 [6]. The 5′ end of the HTT gene comprises a three-nucleotide base sequence, cytosine-adenine-guanine (CAG), which is repeated multiple times

IntechOpen

and codes for the amino acid glutamine. The number of CAG repetitions in a healthy individual varies between 7 and 35. This region of CAG repeats called the trinucleotide repeats varies in length from person to person and may vary in length from generation to generation. The length of the CAG region in the HTT gene is increased due to a hereditary mutation in the HTT gene. The length of the CAG repeats ranges between 36 and 120 in people with HD. Individuals with CAG repeats between 36 and 39 may or may not develop signs of Huntington's disease, whereas individuals with 40 or more repeats always display the characteristic signs and symptoms of Huntington's disease. This expansion of CAG repeats due to the inherited mutation in the HTT gene leads to the production of an unusually long version of huntingtin protein (mHtt) [7]. The mutant huntingtin protein is highly susceptible to cleavage, and this results in the creation of shorter fragments containing polyglutamine expansion. These protein fragments are susceptible to misfolding and aggregation, producing fibrillar aggregates in which non-native polyglutamine strands from different proteins are bonded together by hydrogen bonds. These aggregates share the same basic β-amyloid structure seen in other protein deposition diseases [8]. One of the pathways through which mHtt causes cell death is mitochondrial dysfunction [9]. The impairment of mitochondrial electron transport chain by mHtt increases the level of free radicals and oxidative stress [10]. Following the irrefutable role of oxidative stress and associated neuroinflammation in the pathogenesis of neurodegenerative disorders including Huntington's disease, several exogenous antioxidants were expected to have protective and therapeutic benefits in these degenerative diseases of the brain. But large-scale randomized clinical trials failed to establish any conclusive data to support the hypothesis that exogenous antioxidants could possess neuroprotective or therapeutic benefit in neurodegenerative diseases. Nevertheless, these clinical trials do not refute the fact that oxidative stress and associated neuroinflammation play a key role in the pathogenesis of neurodegenerative diseases. So, it appears logical to stimulate endogenous targets that would reduce oxidative stress and associated neuroinflammation in diseases associated with oxidative stress. Nuclear factor-erythroid-2-related factor 2 (Nrf2) is one such target. Nrf2 is a transcription factor present in the cytoplasm of cells [11]. By upregulating the expression of almost 200 cytoprotective genes, Nrf2 assists cells adapt to inflammation and oxidative stress. Keap1, a repressor protein, controls the level of Nrf2 in the cytoplasm. Keap1 is a cysteine-rich protein that binds to Nrf2 and activates the ubiquitin-proteasome pathway to degrade Nrf2 in the cytoplasm. During oxidative stress, the degradation of Nrf2 by Keap1 is blocked. This results in an increased level of Nrf2 in the cytoplasm of cells. The free Nrf2 moves into the nucleus of cell and increases the transcription of many genes that code for detoxification enzymes and cytoprotective proteins [12]. The potential of Nrf2 to negate oxidative stress and associated neuroinflammation makes it an effective target in the prevention and treatment of Huntington's disease. The focus of this chapter is to review the role of oxidative stress and associated neuroinflammation in Huntington's disease and the potential beneficial effects of Nrf2 activators in Huntington's disease.

2. Oxidative stress in Huntington's disease

Reactive oxygen species (ROS) are highly reactive molecules or molecular fragments formed from oxygen through biochemical reactions that occur during cellular respiration. Reactive oxygen species and reactive nitrogen species exert both beneficial and harmful effects on the living systems [13]. At low to moderate cellular levels, free radicals play a physiological role in destroying the invading pathogenic microorganisms, regulation of signaling pathways and induction of mitogenic response. At high cellular concentrations, free radicals exert a deleterious effect on lipids, proteins, nucleic acids and other cellular structures [14]. In many pathological conditions including Huntington's disease, an increase in the level of free radicals and cellular damage due to free radicals is observed. But it still remains unclear whether free radical induced damage in pathological conditions is a cause or downstream consequence of the underlying pathological process.

3. Antioxidants in Huntington's disease

Antioxidants are substances that are capable of scavenging the free radicals and thereby counteracting the free radical induced oxidative damage and inflammation. There are two classes of antioxidants—enzymatic and non-enzymatic antioxidants. Enzymatic antioxidants include superoxide dismutase (SOD), glutathione peroxidase (Gpx) and catalase (CAT). Ascorbic acid (Vitamin C), carotenoids, α-tocopherol, glutathione (GSH), retinoic acid and flavonoids are examples of non-enzymatic antioxidants. Many of these antioxidants have proven their efficacy in several in vitro and animal models but not in randomized clinical trials. The following table summarizes the findings of the studies that evaluated the efficacy of antioxidants in Huntington's disease (**Table 1**).

Compound	Summary	Reference
α-Tocopherol	α-Tocopherol treatment (50 and 100 mg/kg, p.o.) significantly reversed the various behavioral, biochemical and mitochondrial alterations in malonic acid treated animals.	[15]
Metalloporphyrins	Metalloporphyrins are a class of metallic antioxidants with a potential to scavenge free radicals. In an *in vitro* model of HD, a manganese porphyrin (manganese (III)tetrakis(4-benzoic acid) porphyrin) reduced significant cell death.	[16]
Grape seed Polyphenolic Extract (GSPE)	GSPE is a natural compound and a strong antioxidant that has been reported to inhibit polyQ aggregation in phaeochromocytoma (PC)-12 cell line.	[17]
Melatonin	In the kainic acid animal model of neurodegeneration, melatonin has shown to be neuroprotective. Melatonin increased neuronal survival while reducing DNA damage. Melatonin therapy effectively reduced the increase in lipid peroxidation, protein carbonyls, and SOD activity inside the striatum in another investigation employing the 3-NP model of HD.	[18, 19]
Selenium	In rats treated with quinolinic acid, selenium reduced lipid peroxidation and enhanced neuronal morphology in the striatum in a dose-dependent manner.	[20]
Pyruvate	Treatment with pyruvate protected against striatal neurodegeneration in a quinolinic acid striatal lesion model of HD. Although smaller dosages had no effect, higher doses had a substantial neuroprotective effect, lowering the striatal lesion area when compared with controls.	[21]
TUDCA	TUDCA (tauroursodeoxycholic acid) is an antioxidant-rich hydrophilic bile acid. In a 3-NP rat model of HD, TUDCA reduced striatal degeneration and improved locomotor and cognitive impairments.	[22]

Compound	Summary	Reference
NAC	Treatment of rats with N-acetylcysteine (NAC), a known glutathione precursor, before exposure to 3-NP protected them from oxidative damage caused by 3-NP, as determined by electron paramagnetic resonance (EPR) and protein carbonyl analyzes on a Western blot. Furthermore, NAC therapy prior to 3-NP delivery reduced striatal lesion volumes considerably.	[23]
Lycopene	In a 3-NP induced mouse model of HD, lycopene, a carotenoid pigment and phytochemical naturally found in fruits and vegetables, decreased oxidative stress markers and improved behavior.	[24]
α-Tocopherol	In patients with mild to moderate HD symptoms, a year-long placebo-controlled, double-blind research was conducted. Although α-tocopherol had no effect on neurologic or neuropsychiatric symptoms in the overall therapy group, post hoc analysis revealed that it had a substantial effect on neurologic symptoms in HD patients early in the disease's course.	[25]
Idebenone	A double-blind, placebo-controlled trial of idebenone in 92 HD patients was performed and no effect on primary outcome measures when compared with placebo controls were detected.	[26]

Table 1.
List of antioxidants studied in Huntington's disease.

4. PGC1α-mediated oxidative stress in Huntington's disease

The peroxisome proliferator-activated receptor co-activator-1α (PGC1α) is a transcriptional regulator present in tissues that have a high energy demand such as the brain, liver, cardiomyocytes, adipocytes, skeletal muscles and the kidneys [27, 28]. PGC1α plays a key role in mitochondrial biogenesis, metabolism, peroxisomal remodeling and detoxification of reactive oxygen species [29]. An important and effective mechanism through which PGC1α confers neuroprotection is by its antioxidant activity. Oxidative stress is suppressed by PGC1α by inducing the formation of antioxidant enzymes such as SOD1, SOD2, Gpx-1 and mitochondrial uncoupling proteins [30]. PGC1α also regulates the expression of SIRT3 in mitochondria and SIRT3 in turn activates SOD2 via deacetylation and reduces the level of reactive oxygen species [31, 32]. In short, PGC1α plays a key role in improving mitochondrial function, biogenesis, expression of antioxidant enzymes and amelioration of oxidative stress induced neuronal damage. A deficiency of PGC1α in the brain affects the integrity of mitochondrial structure and increases the level of reactive oxygen species leading to cellular senescence and disorders related to aging [33]. PGC1α expression has been found to be disturbed in neurodegenerative diseases such as Huntington's disease, Parkinson's disease and multiple sclerosis, resulting in mitochondrial abnormalities and elevated ROS levels [34–36]. Therapeutic agents that can activate endogenous antioxidant systems such as Nrf2/ARE pathway leading to increased expression of antioxidant enzymes hold great promise as neuroprotective agents in Huntington's disease. Transcriptional modification of Nrf2 pathway, therefore, is considered an excellent approach to counteract the oxidative stress-mediated neuronal damage in Huntington's disease.

In Huntington's disease, mHtt causes an increase in oxidative stress mediated by PGC1α. mHtt binds to the promoter sequence of PGC1α and reduces the transcriptional level of PGC1α [37]. mHtt also supresses the expression of mitochondrial uncoupling proteins and antioxidant enzymes by direct binding and inactivation of PGC1α [30].

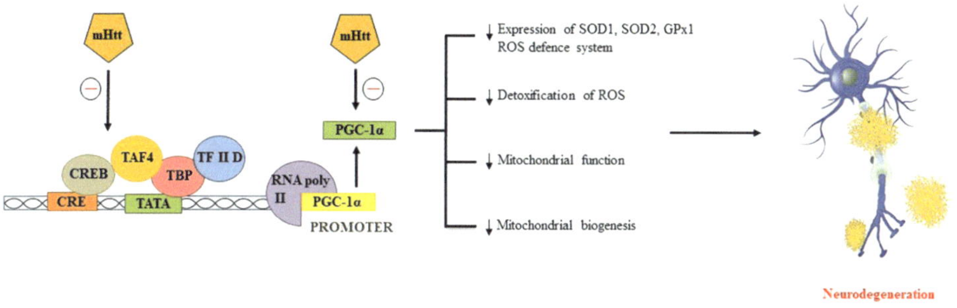

Figure 1.
PGC1α-mediated oxidative stress in Huntington's disease.

mHtt disrupts the balance between mitochondrial fission-fusion process by interfering with the function of Drp1 [38]. mHtt induces leakage of calcium ions through the calcium channel ryanodine receptors, further resulting in opening of the mitochondrial permeability transition pore (mPTP), which contributes to mitochondrial oxidative stress [39]. PGC-1α transcription and activity impact the enzyme system that combats reactive oxygen species (ROS). As a result, ROS defense genes such as SOD1, SOD2 and glutathione peroxidase (GPx1) are downregulated, resulting in increased oxidative damage and neuronal death in Huntington's disease (**Figure 1**).

5. Microgliosis, oxidative stress and associated neuroinflammation in Huntington's disease

Microglial cells are the resident immune cells of the central nervous system (CNS) and make up between 10 and 15% of all glial cells in the brain. Microglial cells develop from pro-erythromyeloid progenitor cells in the yolk sac during embryogenesis and go through three stages of development: early, pre and adult microglia. They then migrate into the CNS, using white matter tracts as guiding structures, until the blood-brain barrier is formed. Microglial cells, once inside the CNS, multiply and disseminate evenly to various regions of the brain and maintain a constant population through self-renewal [40]. Microglial cells have numerous slender and elongated processes branching from the small oval-shaped body, which makes them appear ramified. However, when the brain is exposed to potential dangers such as infection, trauma or other factors, these cells lose their branches and take on an amoeboid shape. Microglial cells in the CNS are involved in the establishment and remodeling of neural circuits, protection and repair of the brain, phagocytosis of apoptotic cells in the developing brain, organization of synapses, neurogenesis, control of myelin turnover, control of neuronal excitability and programmed cell death [41, 42]. Homeostatic microglial cells interact with practically every component of the CNS to maintain homeostasis, development and repair by continuously monitoring ongoing actions in the brain. When microglial cells detect a threat to the CNS's homeostasis, they become activated and produce a variety of cytokines and pro-inflammatory mediators to neutralize the threat. Although this acute response of microglial cells is protective and necessary for maintaining CNS homeostasis, over-activation of microglial cells has been linked to a variety of neurodegenerative diseases [43]. Microglial cells, after activation, release pro-inflammatory mediators and several cytokines that lead to severe oxidative stress and neuroinflammation. According to recent research, activated microglial cells release cytokines and pro-inflammatory mediators, which are the main contributors to neuroinflammation in neurodegenerative diseases [44–46].

A significant increase in microgliosis has been observed in the autopsied brains of the patients with Huntington's disease compared with the controls. Accumulation of glial cells has been observed in all grades of Huntington's disease, and the density of microglial cells finely correlates with the degree of neuronal loss [47, 48]. A significant activation of microglial cells in the regions of the brain affected by Huntington's disease has been reported in an *in vivo* positron emission tomography [49, 50]. In Huntington's disease, microglial cells are activated by mHtt protein, and activated glial cells cause degeneration of neurons in the striatal region of the brain by releasing a variety of proinflammatory cytokines and free radicals [51, 52].

6. Structure of Nrf2

The Nrf2 protein contains 6 highly conserved regions called Nrf2-ECH (Neh) homology domains. The first domain (Neh1) carries the CNC-bZIP domain that mediates heterodimerization with Maf (musculoaponeurotic fibrosarcoma oncogene homolog) proteins. Two degrons called DLG and ETGF, present in the second domain (Neh2) specifically bind to Keap1 protein that leads to degradation of Nrf2 [53]. The third domain (Neh3) is considered to improve the stability of Nrf2 and also acts as the transactivation domain. The fourth (Neh4) and fifth (Neh5) domains of Nrf2 also act as transactivation domains by binding to cAMP response Element Binding Protein (CREB). The sixth domain (Neh6) plays a role in the degradation of Nrf2 by E3 ubiquitin ligase [54].

7. Structure of Keap1

'Kelch-like ECH-associated protein 1(Keap 1) is a protein that interacts with Nrf2 leading to degradation of Nrf2. Keap1 is a protein of BTB-Kelch family, composed of four domains. The N-terminal domain—Broad complex, Tramtrack and Bric a Bric (BTB) control homodimerization of Keap 1 and its interaction with cul3. This domain also contains Cys-151 residue that plays an important role in sensing oxidative stress. The second domain called the intervening region (IVR) domain contains Cys-273 and Cys-288. These two cysteine residues play a secondary role in sensing oxidative stress. The third domain, double glycine repeat (DGR) and the fourth domain, C-terminal region (CTR) binds to ETGE and DLG motifs of Nrf2 and causing its degradation (**Figure 2**) [54].

8. Mechanism of action of Nrf2 activators

Nrf2 is a transcription factor that regulates the expression of many antioxidant enzymes, phase I and phase II enzymes and several anti-inflammatory mediators. Nrf2 acts as an important defense mechanism in the neurons and glial cells against oxidative stress, neuroinflammation and other pathological insults. Nrf2 dysregulation has been reported in many oxidative-stress-related diseases such as Huntington's

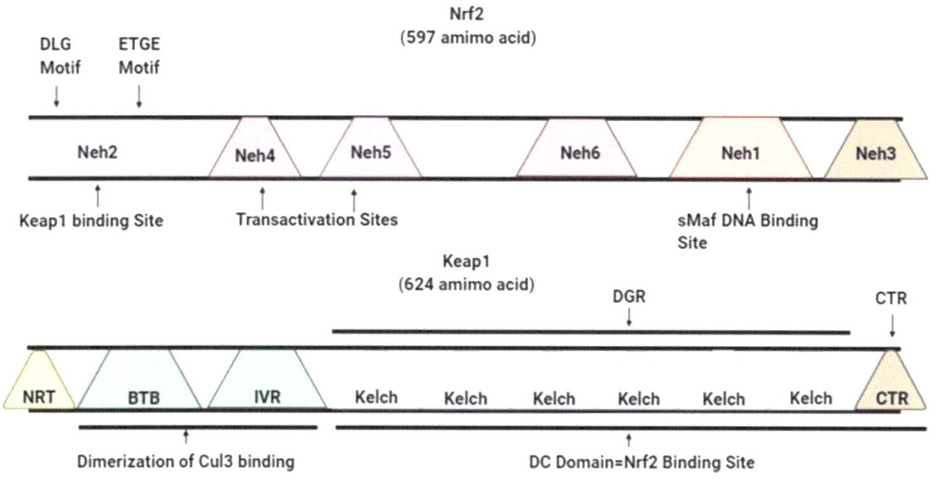

Figure 2.
Structure of Nrf2 and Keap1.

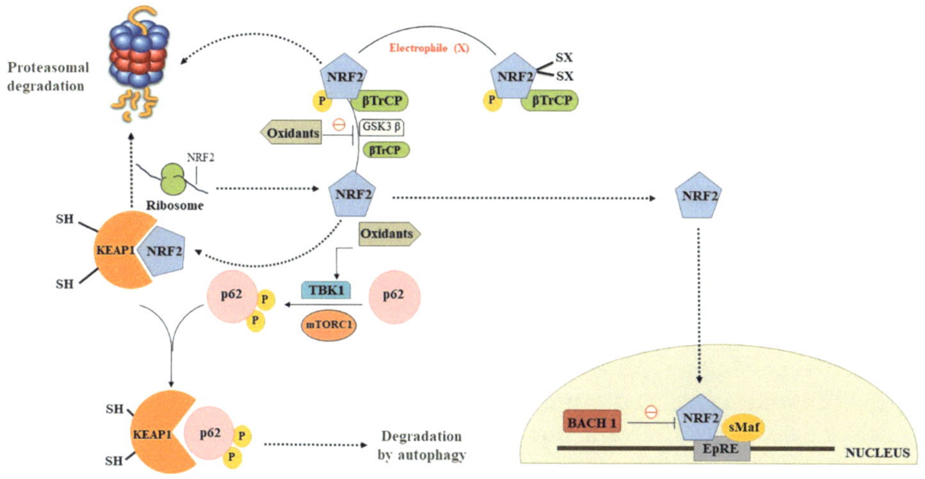

Figure 3.
Mechanism of action of Nrf2 activators.

disease [54]. This makes Nrf2 activators excellent agents to increase antioxidant capacity, decrease neuroinflammation and alleviate pathology in Huntington's disease (**Figure 3**).

Nuclear factor E2-related factor (Nrf2) is a transcription factor composed of 605 amino acids that controls the expression of as many as 200 genes [55–57]. The proteins encoded by Nrf2 genes are control several functions such as anti-inflammation, antioxidant defense, apoptosis, detoxification, removal of oxidized protein by proteasome and DNA repair [58–60]. In physiological conditions, the half-life of Nrf2 is very short (<20 minutes) as it is continuously degraded by Kelch-like ECH-associated protein 1 (Keap 1) [61]. Keap 1 is a regulatory protein that regulates the levels of Nrf2 in the cytoplasm of cell. In basal conditions, the Neh2 domain of Nrf2 binds to the β-barrel structure of Keap-1. This is followed by binding of Cullin-3 to Keap-1-Nrf2 complex, and this results in the formation of ubiquitin 3-ligase complex. The ubiquitin 3-ligase complex bins to many ubiquitin molecules resulting in polyubiquitination of Nrf2, which serves as a signal for proteasomal degradation [62]. Keap-1 contain a lot of cysteines in their structure and the free sulfhydryl (−SH) of cysteine help keap-1 to act as sensors of oxidative stress. During oxidative stress, electrophiles alkylate keap-1 and prevent keap-1 from degrading Nrf2. This leads to accumulation of recently synthesized Nrf2 that increases the antioxidant potential by promoting the transcription of antioxidant and detoxifying genes. In an alternative pathway, Nrf2 is degraded by phosphorylation by glycogen synthase kinase 3β (GSK3β). This degradation of Nrf2 by GSK3β is also blocked by elevated levels of oxidants that leads to accumulation of freshly synthesized Nrf2 [63]. In another pathway, Keap-1 itself is degraded by p62. In this pathway, p62 is phosphorylated by TANK-binding kinase 1 (TBK1) and mechanistic target of rapamycin complex 1 (mTORC1). The phosphorylated p62 makes a complex with keap-1, and this complex is degraded by autophagy in cells [63]. Activation of all these pathways by oxidants leads to accumulation of newly synthesized Nrf2. Nrf2 escapes breakdown into the nucleus and forms heterodimers with sMaf (Nrf2/sMaf). In the nucleus, the activity of Nrf2 is negatively regulated by BACH-1, which competes with Nrf2 to form heterodimers with sMaf [63]. The binding of Nrf2/sMaf to antioxidant response elements promotes the expression of as many as 200 cytoprotective genes.

9. Nrf2 activators in Huntington's disease

Minhee Jang et al. have reported that gintonin, a ginseng-derived lysophosphatidic acid receptor ligand, alleviated the severity of neurological impairment and lethality following 3-nitropropionic acid treatment in laboratory animals through activation of Nrf2. The authors of this study conclude that gintonin might be an innovative therapeutic candidate to treat HD-like syndromes because of its potential to activate Nrf2 and decrease oxidative stress and neuroinflammation [64]. A similar study evaluated the effect of Sulforaphane in animal model of 3-NP acid-induced Huntington's disease. The study revealed that pre-treatment with sulforaphane activated Nrf2 in animals and decreased the formation of a lesion area, neuronal death, succinate dehydrogenase activity, apoptosis, microglial activation and expression of inflammatory mediators, including tumor necrosis factor-alpha, interleukin (IL)-1β, IL-6, inducible nitric oxide synthase and cyclooxygenase-2 in the striatum after 3-NP treatment [65]. Similarly, curcumin is also reported to have beneficial effects in HD via activation of Nrf2 [66]. D. Moretti et al. have reported that compound 2, a covalent KEAP1 binder, demonstrated an ability to stimulate the expression of genes known to be regulated by Nrf2 in neurons and astrocytes separated from wild-type rat, wild-type mouse and zQ175 (an HD mouse model) embryo [67].

10. Challenges facing Nrf2 activators

One of the main challenges associated with Nrf2 activators is achieving effective therapeutic concentrations as these agents are metabolized faster leading to a low bioavailability in distal organs [68–70]. The second concern with Nrf2 activators is lack of selectivity as these agents have been reported to act on other signaling pathways and affect associated physiological processes. For instance, sulforophane, a widely reported Nrf2 activator, suppresses the activation of inflammosome [71, 72] and causes cell arrest [73]. Nrf2 activators have been reported to promote the development of cancer [74–76] and development of resistance to anti-cancer drugs [77–80].

11. Current status of Nrf2 activators

Oxidative stress plays a significant role in pathophysiology of numerous diseases. Initially, exogenous antioxidants were expected to have a protective and therapeutic role in the management of diseases associated with oxidative stress. But randomized clinical trials failed to find any significant therapeutic benefits of exogenous antioxidants. This unexpected outcome led to a search for endogenous targets that would enhance the antioxidant potential of the cells and tissues to prevent oxidative stress-induced damage. This quest for an endogenous antioxidant target led to the discovery of Nrf2 in the year 1994 [81]. Five years later, in 1999, it was discovered that the levels of Nrf2 in the cytoplasm are controlled by a negative regulator, Keap-1 [61]. In recent years, many potential Nrf2 activators are in pre-clinical and different stages of clinical trials for various diseases associated with oxidative stress. **Table 2** provides a list of potential Nrf2 activators in clinical trials and possible indications.

Compound	Indications	Clinical trial	Reference
Bordoxolone methyl	Pulmonary arterial hypertension Alport syndrome Type I diabetes, Polycystic kidney disease Nephropathy Glomerulosclerosis	II/III	[82]
Omaveloxolone	Friedreich's ataxia	II	[82]
Bordoxolone methyl	Type II diabetes Chronic kidney disease		[82]
ALK8700	Multiple Sclerosis	III	[82]
OT551	Dry eye macular degeneration.	II	[82]
CXA10	Primary focal segmental glomerulosclerosis Pulmonary arterial hypertension	II	[82]
XP23829	Psoriasis	II	[82]
SFX-01	Subarachnoid hemorrhage ER+ metastatic breast cancer (in combination with tamoxifen and fulvestrant)	II	[82]
Compound A	Chronic obstructive pulmonary disease	Preclinical	[83]
KEAP1 inhibitors	Parkinson's disease Amyotrophic lateral sclerosis	Preclinical	[82]
M102	Amyotrophic lateral sclerosis Neurodegenerative diseases.	Preclinical	[82]
RS9	Retinovascular disease	Preclinical	[84]
TFM735	Progression of experimental autoimmune encephalitis	Preclinical	[85]

Compound	Indications	Clinical trial	Reference
CAT4001	Friedreich ataxia Amyotrophic lateral sclerosis	Preclinical	[82]
ML334	Type II diabetes Chronic obstructive pulmonary disease.	Preclinical	[86]
HPP971	Blood, lung, eye, kidney and bone diseases.	Preclinical	[87]
VCB101	Multiple Sclerosis	Preclinical	[82]
VCB102	Psoriasis	Preclinical	[82]
Sulforaphane	Schizophrenia Atopic asthmatics Chronic obstructive pulmonary disease Melanoma Prostate cancer Breast cancer Lung cancer Diabetes Mellitus Rhinitis *Helicobacter pylori* infection	Different stages of clinical trials	[88]
Curcumin	Acute kidney injury Schizophrenia Type 2 diabetes Chronic kidney disease Alzheimer's disease Crohn's disease Prostate cancer Major depression abdominal aortic aneurysm	—	[88]
ITH12674	Brain ischemia	Preclinical	[88]
Resveratrol	Type 2 diabetes Colon cancer Chronic Obstructive Pulmonary Disease Endometriosis Alzheimer's disease Huntington's disease Chronic renal insufficiency Non-ischemic cardiomyopathy Non-alcoholic fatty liver Friedreich ataxia	Clinical	[88]
CXA-10	Acute kidney injury Pulmonary arterial hypertension Primary focal segmental glomerulosclerosis.	I II	[88]
RTA 408	Topical application	—	[89]
Fimasartan	Unilateral ureteral obstruction	Preclinical	[90]
Artesunate	Sepsis induced lung injury	Preclinical	[91]
Isovitexin	LPS-induced acute lung injury	—	[92]
Sappanone A	LPS-induced mortality	Preclinical	[93]
Bixin	Ventilation injured lung injury	Preclinical	[94, 95]
Eriodictyol	Cisplatin-induced kidney injury	Preclinical	[96]
Anthocyanin	Atherosclerosis	—	

Table 2.
List of current Nrf2 activators.

12. Conclusion

As free radicals-induced oxidative stress has been proven to play a major role in the pathogenesis of several diseases, it is quintessential to develop antioxidant therapies to negate oxidative stress-induced damage. The initial expectation that exogenous antioxidants such as vitamin E, vitamin C might have a therapeutic benefit in diseases associated with oxidative stress has failed to find any significant beneficial proof in randomized clinical trials. So, it is time to find agents that activate endogenous antioxidant mechanisms such as Nrf2. Nrf2 activators might offer a beneficial action in diseases associated with oxidative stress such as Huntington's disease.

Acknowledgements

The authors would like to thank the Department of Science and Technology—Fund for Improvement of Science and Technology Infrastructure in Universities and Higher Educational Institutions (DST-FIST), New Delhi, for their infrastructure support to our department. We acknowledge the generous research infrastructure and support from JSS College of Pharmacy, JSS Academy of Higher Education & Research, Rocklands, Ooty, The Nilgiris, Tamil Nadu, India.

Author details

Saravanan Jayaram*, Praveen Thaggikuppe Krishnamurthy, Meghana Joshi and Vishnu Kumar
Department of Pharmacology, JSS College of Pharmacy, JSS Academy of Higher Education and Research, Ooty, Tamil Nadu, India

*Address all correspondence to: getsarwan@gmail.com

References

[1] McGarry A, Biglan K, Marshall F. Huntington's disease: Clinical features, disease mechanisms, and management. In: Rosenberg's Molecular and Genetic Basis of Neurological and Psychiatric Disease. London, UK: Elsevier; 2020. pp. 135-145. DOI: 10.1016/b978-0-12-813866-3.00009-6

[2] Cisbani G, Cicchetti F. An in vitro perspective on the molecular mechanisms underlying mutant huntingtin protein toxicity. Cell Death and Disease. 2012;**3**. DOI: 10.1038/cddis.2012.121

[3] Saavedra A, García-Díaz Barriga G, Pérez-Navarro E, Alberch J. Huntington's disease: Novel therapeutic perspectives hanging in the balance. Expert Opinion on Therapeutic Targets. 2018;**22**:385-399. DOI: 10.1080/14728222.2018.1465930

[4] Munoz-Sanjuan I, Bates GP. The importance of integrating basic and clinical research toward the development of new therapies for Huntington disease. Journal of Clinical Investigation. 2011;**121**:476-483. DOI: 10.1172/JCI45364

[5] Franco-Iborra S, Plaza-Zabala A, Montpeyo M, Sebastian D, Vila M, Martinez-Vicente M. Mutant HTT (huntingtin) impairs mitophagy in a cellular model of Huntington disease. Autophagy. 2021;**17**:672-689. DOI: 10.1080/15548627.2020.1728096

[6] MacDonald ME, Ambrose CM, Duyao MP, Myers RH, Lin C, Srinidhi L, et al. A novel gene containing a trinucleotide repeat that is expanded and unstable on Huntington's disease chromosomes. Cell. 1993;**72**:971-983. DOI: 10.1016/0092-8674(93)90585-E

[7] McColgan P, Tabrizi SJ. Huntington's disease: A clinical review. European Journal of Neurology. 2018;**25**:24-34. DOI: 10.1111/ene.13413

[8] Rubinsztein DC, Carmichael J. Huntington's disease: Molecular basis of neurodegeneration. Expert Reviews in Molecular Medicine. 2003;**5**:1-21. DOI: 10.1017/S1462399403006549

[9] Liu Z, Zhou T, Ziegler AC, Dimitrion P, Zuo L. Oxidative stress in neurodegenerative diseases: From molecular mechanisms to clinical applications. Oxidative Medicine and Cellular Longevity. 2017;**2017**. DOI: 10.1155/2017/2525967

[10] Kumar A, Ratan RR. Oxidative stress and Huntington's disease: The good, the bad, and the ugly. Journal of Huntington's Disease. 2016;**5**:217-237. DOI: 10.3233/JHD-160205

[11] Gazaryan IG, Thomas B. The status of Nrf2-based therapeutics: Current perspectives and future prospects. Neural Regeneration Research. 2016;**11**:1708-1711. DOI: 10.4103/1673-5374.194706

[12] Tkachev VO, Menshchikova EB, Zenkov NK. Mechanism of the Nrf2/Keap1/ARE signaling system. Biochemistry (Moscow). 2011;**76**:407-422. DOI: 10.1134/S0006297911040031

[13] di Meo S, Venditti P. Evolution of the knowledge of free radicals and other oxidants. Oxidative Medicine and Cellular Longevity. 2020;**2020**. DOI: 10.1155/2020/9829176

[14] Valko M, Leibfritz D, Moncol J, Cronin MTD, Mazur M, Telser J. Free radicals and antioxidants in normal physiological functions and human disease. International Journal of Biochemistry and Cell Biology.

2007;**39**:44-84. DOI: 10.1016/j.biocel.2006.07.001

[15] Kalonia H, Kumar P, Kumar A. Targeting oxidative stress attenuates malonic acid induced Huntington like behavioral and mitochondrial alterations in rats. European Journal of Pharmacology. 2010;**634**:46-52. DOI: 10.1016/J.EJPHAR.2010.02.031

[16] Petersén Å, Castilho RF, Hansson O, Wieloch T, Brundin P. Oxidative stress, mitochondrial permeability transition and activation of caspases in calcium ionophore A23187-induced death of cultured striatal neurons. Brain Research. 2000;**857**:20-29. DOI: 10.1016/S0006-8993(99)02320-3

[17] Wang J, Pfleger CM, Friedman L, Vittorino R, Zhao W, Qian X, et al. Potential application of grape derived polyphenols in Huntington's disease. Translational Neuroscience. 2010;**1**:95-100. DOI: 10.2478/V10134-010-0022-Y

[18] Túnez I, Montilla P, Muñoz MDC, Feijóo M, Salcedo M. Protective effect of melatonin on 3-nitropropionic acid-induced oxidative stress in synaptosomes in an animal model of Huntington's disease. Journal of Pineal Research. 2004;**37**:252-256. DOI: 10.1111/J.1600-079X.2004.00163.X

[19] Uz T, Giusti P, Franceschini D, Kharlamov A, Manev H. Protective effect of melatonin against hippocampal DNA damage induced by intraperitoneal administration of kainate to rats. Neuroscience. 1996;**73**:631-636. DOI: 10.1016/0306-4522(96)00155-8

[20] Santamaría A, Salvatierra-Sánchez R, Vázquez-Román B, Santiago-López D, Villeda-Hernández J, Galván-Arzate S, et al. Protective effects of the antioxidant selenium on quinolinic acid-induced neurotoxicity in rats: In vitro and in vivo studies. Journal of Neurochemistry. 2003;**86**:479-488. DOI: 10.1046/J.1471-4159.2003.01857.X

[21] Ryu JK, Kim SU, McLarnon JG. Neuroprotective effects of pyruvate in the quinolinic acid rat model of Huntington's disease. Experimental Neurology. 2003;**183**:700-704. DOI: 10.1016/S0014-4886(03)00214-0

[22] Keene CD, Rodrigues CMP, Eich T, Linehan-Stieers C, Abt A, Kren BT, et al. A bile acid protects against motor and cognitive deficits and reduces striatal degeneration in the 3-nitropropionic acid model of Huntington's disease. Experimental Neurology. 2001;**171**:351-360. DOI: 10.1006/EXNR.2001.7755

[23] la Fontaine MA, Geddes JW, Banks A, Allan BD. Effect of exogenous and endogenous antioxidants on 3-nitropionic acid-induced in vivo oxidative stress and striatal lesions: Insights into Huntington's disease. Journal of Neurochemistry. 2000;**75**:1709-1715. DOI: 10.1046/J.1471-4159.2000.0751709.X

[24] Kumar P, Kumar A. Effect of lycopene and epigallocatechin-3-gallate against 3-nitropropionic acid induced cognitive dysfunction and glutathione depletion in rat: A novel nitric oxide mechanism. Food and Chemical Toxicology: An International Journal Published for the British Industrial Biological Research Association. 2009;**47**:2522-2530. DOI: 10.1016/J.FCT.2009.07.011

[25] Peyser CE, Folstein M, Chase GA, Starkstein S, Brandt J, Cockrell JR, et al. Trial of d-alpha-tocopherol in Huntington's disease. The American Journal of Psychiatry. 1995;**152**:1771-1775. DOI: 10.1176/AJP.152.12.1771

[26] Ranen NG, Peyser CE, Coyle JT, Bylsma FW, Sherr M, Day L, et al.

A controlled trial of idebenone in Huntington's disease. Movement Disorders : Official Journal of the Movement Disorder Society. 1996;**11**: 549-554. DOI: 10.1002/MDS.870110510

[27] Tritos NA, Mastaitis JW, Kokkotou EG, Puigserver P, Spiegelman BM, Maratos-Flier E. Characterization of the peroxisome proliferator activated receptor coactivator 1 alpha (PGC 1alpha) expression in the murine brain. Brain Research. 2003;**961**:255-260. DOI: 10.1016/S0006-8993(02)03961-6

[28] Esterbauer H, Oberkofler H, Krempler F, Patsch W. Human peroxisome proliferator activated receptor gamma coactivator 1 (PPARGC1) gene: CDNA sequence, genomic organization, chromosomal localization, and tissue expression. Genomics. 1999;**62**:98-102. DOI: 10.1006/GENO.1999.5977

[29] Puigserver P, Spiegelman BM. Peroxisome proliferator-activated receptor-gamma coactivator 1 alpha (PGC-1 alpha): Transcriptional coactivator and metabolic regulator. Endocrine Reviews. 2003;**24**:78-90. DOI: 10.1210/ER.2002-0012

[30] St-Pierre J, Drori S, Uldry M, Silvaggi JM, Rhee J, Jäger S, et al. Suppression of reactive oxygen species and neurodegeneration by the PGC-1 transcriptional coactivators. Cell. 2006;**127**:397-408. DOI: 10.1016/J.CELL.2006.09.024

[31] Qiu X, Brown K, Hirschey MD, Verdin E, Chen D. Calorie restriction reduces oxidative stress by SIRT3-mediated SOD2 activation. Cell Metabolism. 2010;**12**:662-667. DOI: 10.1016/J.CMET.2010.11.015

[32] Ozden O, Park SH, Kim HS, Jiang H, Coleman MC, Spitz DR, et al. Acetylation of MnSOD directs enzymatic activity responding to cellular nutrient status or oxidative stress. Aging. 2011;**3**:102-107. DOI: 10.18632/AGING.100291

[33] Kim SB, Heo JI, Kim H, Kim KS. Acetylation of PGC1α by histone deacetylase 1 downregulation is implicated in radiation-induced senescence of brain endothelial cells. The Journals of Gerontology Series A, Biological Sciences and Medical Sciences. 2019;**74**:787-793. DOI: 10.1093/GERONA/GLY167

[34] Witte ME, Nijland PG, Drexhage JAR, Gerritsen W, Geerts D, van het Hof B, et al. Reduced expression of PGC-1α partly underlies mitochondrial changes and correlates with neuronal loss in multiple sclerosis cortex. Acta Neuropathologica. 2013;**125**:231-243. DOI: 10.1007/S00401-012-1052-Y

[35] Che HVB, Metzger S, Portal E, Deyle C, Riess O, Nguyen HP. Localization of sequence variations in PGC-1 influence their modifying effect in Huntington disease. Molecular Neurodegeneration. 2011;**6**:1-7. DOI: 10.1186/1750-1326-6-1/TABLES/6

[36] Pacelli C, de Rasmo D, Signorile A, Grattagliano I, di Tullio G, D'Orazio A, et al. Mitochondrial defect and PGC-1α dysfunction in parkin-associated familial Parkinson's disease. Biochimica et Biophysica Acta. 1812;**2011**:1041-1053. DOI: 10.1016/J.BBADIS.2010.12.022

[37] Chaturvedi RK, Hennessey T, Johri A, Tiwari SK, Mishra D, Agarwal S, et al. Transducer of regulated creb-binding proteins (TORCs) transcription and function is impaired in Huntington's disease. Human Molecular Genetics. 2012;**21**:3474-3488. DOI: 10.1093/hmg/dds178

[38] Shirendeb U, Reddy AP, Manczak M, Calkins MJ, Mao P, Tagle DA, et al.

Abnormal mitochondrial dynamics, mitochondrial loss and mutant huntingtin oligomers in Huntington's disease: Implications for selective neuronal damage. Human Molecular Genetics. 2011;**20**:1438-1455. DOI: 10.1093/HMG/DDR024

[39] Suzuki M, Nagai Y, Wada K, Koike T. Calcium leak through ryanodine receptor is involved in neuronal death induced by mutant huntingtin. Biochemical and Biophysical Research Communications. 2012;**429**:18-23. DOI: 10.1016/J. BBRC.2012.10.107

[40] Matcovitch-Natan O, Winter DR, Giladi A, Aguilar SV, Spinrad A, Sarrazin S, et al. Microglia development follows a stepwise program to regulate brain homeostasis. Science. 2016;**353**. DOI: 10.1126/science.aad8670

[41] Bachiller S, Jiménez-ferrer I, Paulus A, Yang Y, Swanberg M, Hayley S, et al. Microglia in neurological diseases: A road map to brain-disease dependent-inflammatory response. Frontiers in Cellular Neuroscience. 2018;**12**:1-17. DOI: 10.3389/fncel.2018.00488

[42] Li Q, Barres BA. Microglia and macrophages in brain homeostasis and disease. Nature Publishing Group. 2017;**18**:225-242. DOI: 10.1038/ nri.2017.125

[43] Ginhoux F, Lim S, Hoeffel G, Low D, Huber T, Cuadros MA. Origin and differentiation of microglia. Frontiers in Cellular Neuroscience. 2013;7:1-14. DOI: 10.3389/ fncel.2013.00045

[44] Liu C, Wang X, Liu C, Zhang H, Di L, Mannelli C. Pharmacological targeting of microglial activation: New therapeutic approach. Frontiers in Cellular Neuroscience 2019;**13**:1-19. DOI: 10.3389/fncel.2019.00514

[45] Galloway DA, Phillips AEM, Owen DRJ, Moore CS, Moore CS. Phagocytosis in the brain : Homeostasis and disease. Frontiers in Immunology. 2019;**10**:1-15. DOI: 10.3389/fimmu. 2019.00790

[46] Bachiller S, Jiménez-Ferrer I, Paulus A, Yang Y, Swanberg M, Deierborg T, et al. Microglia in neurological diseases: A road map to brain-disease dependent-inflammatory response. Frontiers in Cellular Neuroscience. 2018;**12**:488. DOI: 10.3389/FNCEL.2018.00488/BIBTEX

[47] Sapp E, Kegel KB, Aronin N, Hashikawa T, Uchiyama Y, Tohyama K, et al. Early and progressive accumulation of reactive microglia in the Huntington disease brain. Journal of Neuropathology & Experimental Neurology. 2001;**60**:161-172. DOI: 10.1093/JNEN/60.2.161

[48] Myers RH, Vonsattel JP, Paskevich PA, Kiely DK, Stevens TJ, Cupples LA, et al. Decreased neuronal and increased oligodendroglial densities in Huntington's disease caudate nucleus. Journal of Neuropathology & Experimental Neurology. 1991;**50**: 729-742. DOI: 10.1097/00005072-199111000-00005

[49] Politis M, Pavese N, Tai YF, Kiferle L, Mason SL, Brooks DJ, et al. Microglial activation in regions related to cognitive function predicts disease onset in Huntington's disease: A multimodal imaging study. Human Brain Mapping. 2011;**32**:258-270. DOI: 10.1002/ HBM.21008

[50] Pavese N, Gerhard A, Tai YF, Ho AK, Turkheimer F, Barker RA, et al. Microglial activation correlates with severity in Huntington disease. Neurology. 2006;**66**:1638-1643. DOI: 10.1212/01.WNL.0000222734. 56412.17

[51] Zhao T, Hong Y, Li S, Li XJ. Compartment-dependent degradation of mutant huntingtin accounts for its preferential accumulation in neuronal processes. The Journal of neuroscience: The official journal of the Society for Neuroscience. 2016;**36**:8317-8328. DOI: 10.1523/JNEUROSCI.0806-16.2016

[52] Li H, Li SH, Johnston H, Shelbourne PF, Li XJ. Amino-terminal fragments of mutant huntingtin show selective accumulation in striatal neurons and synaptic toxicity. Nature Genetics. 2000;**25**:385-389. DOI: 10.1038/78054

[53] Canning P, Sorrell FJ, Bullock AN. Structural basis of Keap1 interactions with Nrf2. Free Radical Biology and Medicine. 2015;**88**:101-107. DOI: 10.1016/j.freeradbiomed.2015.05.034

[54] Deshmukh P, Unni S, Krishnappa G, Padmanabhan B. The Keap1–Nrf2 pathway: Promising therapeutic target to counteract ROS-mediated damage in cancers and neurodegenerative diseases. Biophysical Reviews. 2017;**9**:41-56. DOI: 10.1007/s12551-016-0244-4

[55] Nioi P, Mahon MMC, Itoh K, Yamamoto M, Hayes JD. Identification of a novel Nrf2-regulated antioxidant response element (ARE) in the mouse NAD(P)H: Quinone oxidoreductase 1 gene : Reassessment of the ARE consensus sequence. Biochemical Journal. 2003;**348**:337-348

[56] Friling RS, Bensimon A, Tichauer Y, Daniel V. Xenobiotic-inducible expression of murine glutathione S-transferase Ya subunit gene is controlled by an electrophile-responsive element. Proceedings of the National Academy of Sciences of the United States. 1990;**87**:6258-6262

[57] Banning A, Deubel S, Kluth D, Zhou Z, Brigelius-flohe R. The GI-GPx gene is a target for Nrf2. Molecular & Cellular Biology. 2005;**25**:4914-4923. DOI: 10.1128/MCB.25.12.4914

[58] Kobayashi EH, Suzuki T, Funayama R, Nagashima T, Hayashi M, Sekine H, et al. Nrf2suppressesmacrophageinflammatory response by blocking proinflammatory cytokine transcription. Nature Communications. 2016;**7**:1-14. DOI: 10.1038/ncomms11624

[59] Ushida Y, Talalay P. Sulforaphane accelerates acetaldehyde metabolism by inducing aldehyde dehydrogenases: Relevance to ethanol intolerance. Alcohol and Alcoholism (Oxford, Oxfordshire). 2013;**48**:526-534. DOI: 10.1093/ALCALC/AGT063

[60] Pickering AM, Linder RA, Zhang H, Forman HJ, Davies KJA. Nrf2-dependent induction of proteasome and Pa28αβ regulator are required for adaptation to oxidative stress. The Journal of Biological Chemistry. 2012;**287**:10021. DOI: 10.1074/JBC.M111.277145

[61] Itoh K, Wakabayashi N, Katoh Y, Ishii T, Igarashi K, Engel JD, et al. Keap1 represses nuclear activation of antioxidant responsive elements by Nrf2 through binding to the amino-terminal Neh2 domain. Genes and Development. 1999;**13**:76-86. DOI: 10.1101/gad.13.1.76

[62] Li Y, Paonessa JD, Zhang Y. Mechanism of chemical activation of Nrf2. PLoS One. 2012;**7**. DOI: 10.1371/journal.pone.0035122

[63] Forman HJ, Zhang H. Targeting oxidative stress in disease: Promise and limitations of antioxidant therapy. Nature Reviews Drug Discovery. 2021;**20**:689-709. DOI: 10.1038/s41573-021-00233-1

[64] Jang M, Choi JH, Chang Y, Lee SJ, Nah SY, Cho IH. Gintonin,

a ginseng-derived ingredient, as a novel therapeutic strategy for Huntington's disease: Activation of the Nrf2 pathway through lysophosphatidic acid receptors. Brain, Behavior, and Immunity. 2019;**80**:146-162. DOI: 10.1016/J.BBI.2019.03.001

[65] Jang M, Cho IH. Sulforaphane ameliorates 3-nitropropionic acid-induced striatal toxicity by activating the Keap1-Nrf2-ARE pathway and inhibiting the MAPKs and NF-κB pathways. Molecular Neurobiology. 2016;**53**:2619-2635. DOI: 10.1007/S12035-015-9230-2

[66] Labanca F, Ullah H, Khan H, Milella L, Xiao J, Dajic-Stevanovic Z, et al. Therapeutic and mechanistic effects of curcumin in Huntington's disease. Current Neuropharmacology. 2021;**19**:1007-1018. DOI: 10.2174/1570159X18666200522201123

[67] Moretti D, Tambone S, Cerretani M, Fezzardi P, Missineo A, Sherman LT, et al. NRF2 activation by reversible KEAP1 binding induces the antioxidant response in primary neurons and astrocytes of a Huntington's disease mouse model. Free Radical Biology and Medicine. 2021;**162**:243-254. DOI: 10.1016/J.FREERADBIOMED.2020.10.022

[68] Lipton S, Satoh T. Recent advances in understanding NRF2 as a druggable target: Development of pro-electrophilic and non-covalent NRF2 activators to overcome systemic side effects of electrophilic drugs like dimethyl fumarate. F1000Research. 2017;**6**. DOI: 10.12688/f1000research.12111.1

[69] Couch RD, Browning RG, Honda T, Gribble GW, Wright DL, Sporn MB, et al. Studies on the reactivity of CDDO, a promising new chemopreventive and chemotherapeutic agent: Implications for a molecular mechanism of action. Bioorganic & Medicinal Chemistry Letters. 2005;**15**:2215-2219. DOI: 10.1016/J.BMCL.2005.03.031

[70] Jiang ZY, Lu MC, You QD. Discovery and development of Kelch-like ECH-associated protein 1. Nuclear factor erythroid 2-related factor 2 (KEAP1:NRF2) protein-protein interaction inhibitors: Achievements, challenges, and future directions. Journal of Medicinal Chemistry. 2016;**59**:10837-10858. DOI: 10.1021/acs.jmedchem.6b00586

[71] Greaney AJ, Maier NK, Leppla SH, Moayeri M. Sulforaphane inhibits multiple inflammasomes through an Nrf2-independent mechanism. Journal of Leukocyte Biology. 2016;**99**:189-199. DOI: 10.1189/JLB.3A0415-155RR

[72] Kwon JS, Joung H, Kim YS, Shim YS, Ahn Y, Jeong MH, et al. Sulforaphane inhibits restenosis by suppressing inflammation and the proliferation of vascular smooth muscle cells. Atherosclerosis. 2012;**225**:41-49. DOI: 10.1016/J.ATHEROSCLEROSIS.2012.07.040

[73] Roy SK, Srivastava RK, Shankar S. Inhibition of PI3K/AKT and MAPK/ERK pathways causes activation of FOXO transcription factor, leading to cell cycle arrest and apoptosis in pancreatic cancer. Journal of Molecular Signaling. 2010;**5**. DOI: 10.1186/1750-2187-5-10

[74] Satoh H, Moriguchi T, Takai J, Ebina M, Yamamoto M. Nrf2 prevents initiation but accelerates progression through the kras signaling pathway during lung carcinogenesis. Cancer Research. 2013;**73**:4158-4168. DOI: 10.1158/0008-5472.CAN-12-4499

[75] Wiel C, le Gal K, Ibrahim MX, Jahangir CA, Kashif M, Yao H, et al. BACH1 stabilization by antioxidants

stimulates lung cancer metastasis. Cell. 2019;**178**:330-345.e22. DOI: 10.1016/J.CELL.2019.06.005

[76] Tao S, Rojo de la Vega M, Chapman E, Ooi A, Zhang DD. The effects of NRF2 modulation on the initiation and progression of chemically and genetically induced lung cancer. Molecular Carcinogenesis. 2018;**57**:182. DOI: 10.1002/MC.22745

[77] Homma S, Ishii Y, Morishima Y, Yamadori T, Matsuno Y, Haraguchi N, et al. Nrf2 enhances cell proliferation and resistance to anticancer drugs in human lung cancer. Clinical Cancer Research: An Official Journal of the American Association for Cancer Research. 2009;**15**:3423-3432. DOI: 10.1158/1078-0432.CCR-08-2822

[78] Roh JL, Kim EH, Jang H, Shin D. Nrf2 inhibition reverses the resistance of cisplatin-resistant head and neck cancer cells to artesunate-induced ferroptosis. Redox Biology. 2017;**11**:254-262. DOI: 10.1016/J.REDOX.2016.12.010

[79] Jiang T, Chen N, Zhao F, Wang XJ, Kong B, Zheng W, et al. High levels of Nrf2 determine chemoresistance in type II endometrial cancer. Cancer Research. 2010;**70**:5486-5496. DOI: 10.1158/0008-5472.CAN-10-0713

[80] Shibata T, Kokubu A, Gotoh M, Ojima H, Ohta T, Yamamoto M, et al. Genetic alteration of Keap1 confers constitutive Nrf2 activation and resistance to chemotherapy in gallbladder cancer. Gastroenterology. 2008;**135**. DOI: 10.1053/J.GASTRO.2008.06.082

[81] Moi P, Chant K, Asunis I, Cao A, Kant YWAI. Isolation of NF-E2-related factor 2 (Nrf2), a NF-E2-like basic leucine zipper transcriptional activator that binds to the tandem NF-E2/AP1 repeat of the f-globin locus control region. 1994;**91**:9926-9930

[82] Cuadrado A, Rojo AI, Wells G, Hayes JD, Cousin SP, Rumsey WL, et al. Therapeutic targeting of the NRF2 and KEAP1 partnership in chronic diseases. Nature Reviews Drug Discovery. 2019;**18**:295-317. DOI: 10.1038/s41573-018-0008-x

[83] Davies TG, Wixted WE, Coyle JE, Griffiths-Jones C, Hearn K, McMenamin R, et al. Monoacidic Inhibitors of the Kelch-like ECH-associated protein 1: Nuclear factor erythroid 2-related factor 2 (KEAP1:NRF2) protein-protein interaction with high cell potency identified by fragment-based discovery. Journal of Medicinal Chemistry. 2016;**59**:3991-4006. DOI: 10.1021/acs.jmedchem.6b00228

[84] Nakagami Y, Masuda K, Hatano E, Inoue T, Matsuyama T, Iizuka M, et al. Novel Nrf2 activators from microbial transformation products inhibit blood-retinal barrier permeability in rabbits. British Journal of Pharmacology. 2015;**172**:1237-1249. DOI: 10.1111/bph.12999

[85] Higashi C, Kawaji A, Tsuda N, Hayashi M, Saito R, Furusako S, et al. The novel Nrf2 inducer TFM-735 ameliorates experimental autoimmune encephalomyelitis in mice. European Journal of Pharmacology. 2017;802:1-9. DOI: 10.1016/j.ejphar.2017.02.044

[86] Hu L, Magesh S, Chen L, Wang L, Lewis TA, Chen Y, et al. Discovery of a small-molecule inhibitor and cellular probe of Keap1-Nrf2 protein-protein interaction. Bioorganic & Medicinal Chemistry Letters. 2013;**23**:3039-3043. DOI: 10.1016/j.bmcl.2013.03.013

[87] Attucks OC, Jasmer KJ, Hannink M, Kassis J, Zhong Z, Gupta S, et al. Induction of heme oxygenase I (HMOX1) by HPP-4382: A novel modulator of Bach1 activity. PLoS One.

2014;**9**:e101044. DOI: 10.1371/JOURNAL.PONE.0101044

[88] Robledinos-Antón N, Fernández-Ginés R, Manda G, Cuadrado A. Activators and inhibitors of NRF2: A review of their potential for clinical development. Oxidative Medicine and Cellular Longevity. 2019;**2019**. DOI: 10.1155/2019/9372182

[89] Reisman SA, Goldsberry AR, Lee CI, Grady MLO, Proksch JW, Ward KW, et al. Topical application of RTA 408 lotion activates Nrf2 in human skin and is well- tolerated by healthy human volunteers. BMC Dermatology. 2015;15: 1-11. DOI: 10.1186/s12895-015-0029-7

[90] Kim S, Kim SJ, Yoon HE, Chung S, Choi BS, Park CW, et al. Fimasartan, a novel angiotensin-receptor blocker, protects against renal inflammation and fibrosis in mice with unilateral ureteral obstruction: The possible role of Nrf2. International Journal of Medical Sciences. 2015;**12**:891. DOI: 10.7150/IJMS.13187

[91] Hui CT, Gen JS, Sheng FD, Kang K, Jiang L, Yuan LZ, et al. Artesunate protects against sepsis-induced lung injury via heme oxygenase-1 modulation. Inflammation. 2016;**39**:651-662. DOI: 10.1007/S10753-015-0290-2

[92] Lv H, Yu Z, Zheng Y, Wang L, Qin X, Cheng G, et al. Isovitexin exerts anti-inflammatory and anti-oxidant activities on lipopolysaccharide-induced acute lung injury by inhibiting MAPK and NF-κB and activating HO-1/Nrf2 pathways. International Journal of Biological Sciences. 2016;**12**:72. DOI: 10.7150/IJBS.13188

[93] Lee S, Choi SY, Choo YY, Kim O, Tran PT, Dao CT, et al. Sappanone A exhibits anti-inflammatory effects via modulation of Nrf2 and NF-κB. International Immunopharmacology. 2015;**28**:328-336. DOI: 10.1016/J.INTIMP.2015.06.015

[94] Tao S, Rojo De La Vega M, Quijada H, Wondrak GT, Wang T, Garcia JGN, et al. Bixin protects mice against ventilation-induced lung injury in an NRF2-dependent manner. Scientific Reports. 2016;**6**:1-13. DOI: 10.1038/srep18760

[95] Aboonabi A, Singh I. Chemopreventive role of anthocyanins in atherosclerosis via activation of Nrf2-ARE as an indicator and modulator of redox. Biomedicine & Pharmacotherapy (Biomedecine & Pharmacotherapie). 2015;**72**:30-36. DOI: 10.1016/J.BIOPHA.2015.03.008

[96] Zhu GFA, Guo HJ, Huang YAN, Wu CT, Zhang XF. Eriodictyol , a plant flavonoid , attenuates LPS-induced acute lung injury through its antioxidative and anti-inflammatory activity. Experimental and Therapeutic Medicine. 2015;10(6):2259-2266. DOI: 10.3892/etm.2015.2827